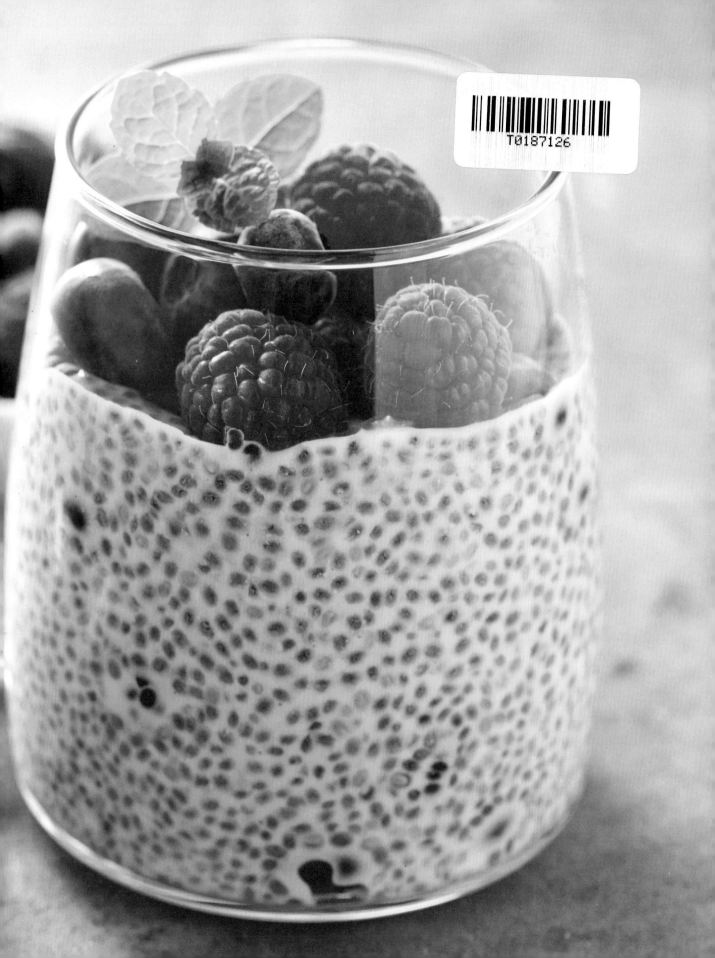

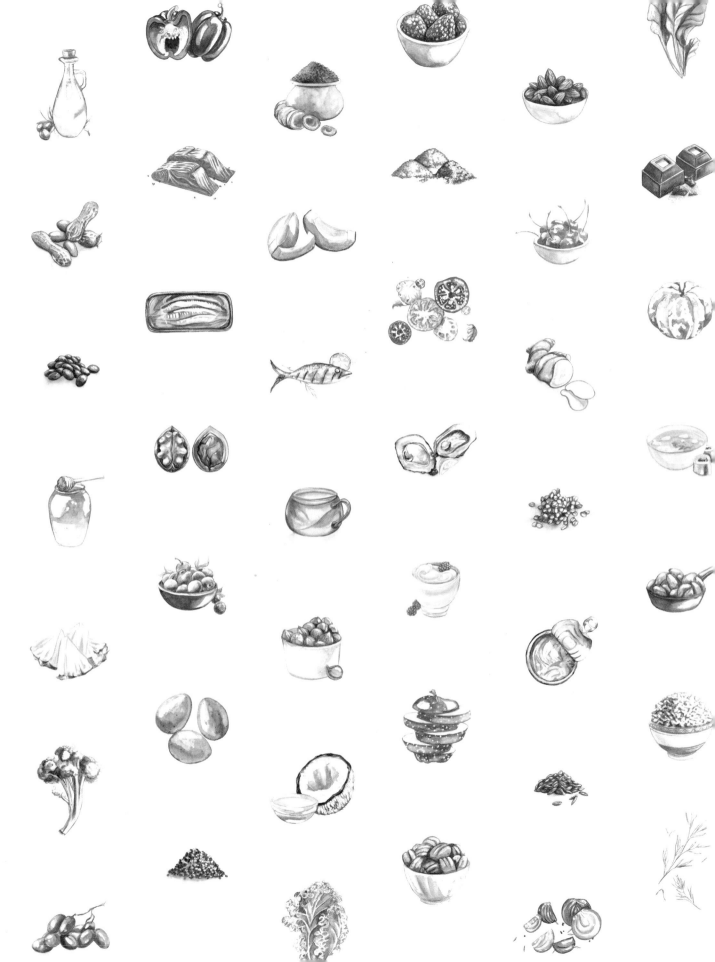

The
Anti-Inflammatory
Cookbook

The Anti-Inflammatory Cookbook

13-Digit ISBN: 978-1-64643-144-1
10-Digit ISBN: 1-64643-144-8

This book may be ordered by mail from the publisher. Please include $5.99 for postage and handling. Please support your local bookseller first!

Books published by Cider Mill Press Book Publishers are available at special discounts for bulk purchases in the United States by corporations, institutions, and other organizations. For more information, please contact the publisher.

Cider Mill Press Book Publishers
"Where good books are ready for press"
PO Box 454
12 Spring Street
Kennebunkport, Maine 04046

Visit us online!
cidermillpress.com

Typography: Brandon Grotesque, Playfair Display

Image Credits: Illustrations courtesy of Cider Mill Press.
All other images used under official license from Shutterstock.com.

Front endpaper image: Overnight Very Berry Chia Seed Pudding, see page 20.

Printed in China
3 4 5 6 7 8 9 0

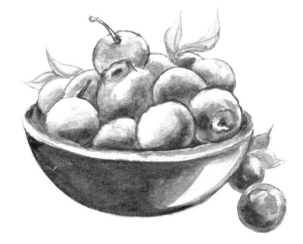

The
Anti-Inflammatory
Cookbook

**BOOST YOUR IMMUNE SYSTEM • DETOX YOUR BODY
OVER 100 RECIPES**

Krissy Carbo, RD

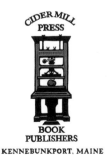

CIDER MILL
PRESS

BOOK
PUBLISHERS
KENNEBUNKPORT, MAINE

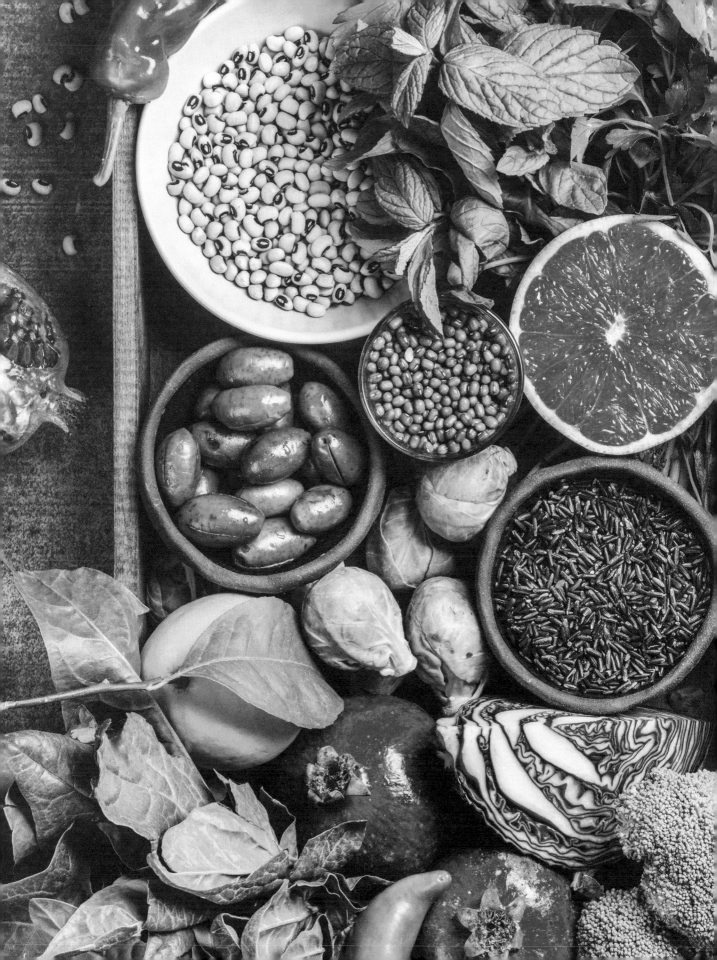

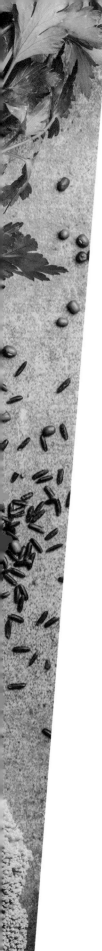

Contents

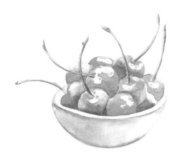

Introduction

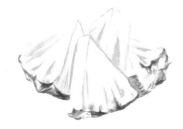

Inflammation is a natural and protective mechanism our immune system possesses to help us heal when we're exposed to harmful pathogens, unknown particles, and physical trauma. Some symptoms of inflammation include fever, body aches, headaches, skin rashes, allergies, swelling, bloating, diarrhea, and fatigue. If you've ever cut yourself, you'll immediately notice pain, redness, and swelling. This is your immune system triggering an acute inflammatory response which increases blood flow to the affected area, thus allowing the appropriate immune cells to arrive quickly and do their job efficiently. Once the bleeding stops and the skin heals, there's no longer an inflammatory immune response. The issue with inflammation starts when the response is no longer acute and it becomes a more persistent inflammatory response. This is known as chronic inflammation, and as research continues to emerge, chronic inflammation is consistently linked to many of the common health complications and diseases we see today, such as hypertension, obesity, diabetes, pre-diabetes, autoimmune disorders, arthritis, allergies, asthma, chronic fatigue, weight-loss resistance, depression, anxiety, and various gastrointestinal issues. So, what causes chronic inflammation?

Most inflammatory triggers come from our environment. The air we breathe, the water we drink, household products we use, stressful events we experience, and the food we eat. Food can be a major source of inflammatory triggers, but it can also serve as a way to protect and heal us from inflammatory triggers as well. An anti-inflammatory diet refers to a way of eating that emphasizes consuming high-quality, nutrient-dense whole foods and minimizing intake of processed foods lacking in nutrients. Eating "whole foods" doesn't mean having to eat only plants or getting all of your food from Whole Foods. It means eating the foods that are closest to their natural state and provide the most amount of essential nutrients per bite. Once your body has the materials it needs to function at its best, you'll see a decrease in inflammatory states that put you at higher risk for chronic disease and health complications. Think about your body as a car. In order for a car to function properly and get you where you need to be, you need to fill it with the correct amount and specific type of gas. If you start filling your car with diesel when it was meant to run on regular gasoline, you're going to run into mechanical issues and you're not going to get very far. The same goes for our bodies. If we feed our bodies food that it wasn't meant to tolerate, like processed convenient foods, our bodies won't be able to get us very far in life without complications and costly visits with a physician.

Standard American diets or Westernized diets that most Americans in this country follow are highly processed and tremendously rich in omega-6 fatty acids and refined sugars—all of which provoke chronic and systemic inflammation within our bodies. Processed foods also tend to lose a lot of their nutritional value during processing. Anti-inflammatory foods give us the most bang for our buck and are packed with crucial nutrients that help our body systems function properly. Foods that are sourced sustainably and are minimally processed support immune system functions, liver detoxification, and gut integrity.

Sourcing your food sustainably is just as important as choosing beneficial foods over nutrient-poor foods. Sourcing sustainably means opting for organic and/or locally grown fruits and vegetables and consuming animal products from animals that were raised in their natural environment (grass-fed cows, pasture-raised chickens, wild-caught fish, humanely raised pork). Conventionally raised fruits and vegetables are grown with the use of pesticides, herbicides, insecticides, and other chemicals that enter our bodies once we eat these foods. Our immune system does not recognize these chemicals, so it sends its army of immune cells to fight and eliminate these foreign particles. This inflammatory response causes damage to the surrounding organ tissues and systems that will then manifest in symptoms of chronic disease.

Buying organic or locally grown produce allows us to avoid these inflammatory triggers. Organic and locally grown produce also tends to have more nutrients that support our health, not just from the vitamins, minerals, antioxidants, phytonutrients, and polyphenol content of the food itself, but from the soil that was used to grow the food. Eating animal products from animals raised in their most natural environment also allows us to take in more quality nutrients. For example, conventionally raised cows are fed a grain-based diet. These grains tend to be high in inflammatory omega-6 fatty acids. Once we eat these animals, the inflammatory fats enter our bodies and wreak havoc. On the other hand, grass-fed cows that are allowed to roam in open pastures are higher in anti-inflammatory omega-3 fatty acids. Omega-3 fatty acids serve many anti-inflammatory functions, making them essential in any anti-inflammatory diet. We need fat. All of our cells are made up of fatty membranes and in order for them to function properly, they need to have a proper structure. Omega-3 fatty acids support our cell membrane structures and protect us from inflammatory triggers. Foods like chia seeds, grass-fed beef, pasture-raised eggs, avocado, avocado oil, hemp seeds, olive oil, grass-fed butter, and wild-caught salmon are rich in omega-3 fatty acids, and you'll find lots of these ingredients in my recipes.

On the subject of sustainably sourced foods, it's important to note that organically grown, pasture-raised, wild-caught, and humanely raised foods are the best option. But if these options are not available to you for whatever reason (they don't work with your budget or they're not available at the store), it is not an excuse to continue to eat processed, refined, nutrient-poor foods. Conventionally raised foods are still far superior to processed foods. If sustainably sourced foods are available to you, great! If not, conventionally raised produce, beef, chicken, and pork still have plenty of anti-inflammatory nutrients that work to support your health, avoid disease, and help your body eliminate toxins, including those associated with conventionally raised foods.

Other anti-inflammatory foods support our gut integrity and intestinal bacteria. Gut health is extremely important in helping avoid inflammation. Much of our immune system lives in our gut, and in order to properly absorb the nutrients from the foods we eat, our gut needs to be in good shape. Avoiding highly processed, sugar-laden foods also keeps populations of harmful gut bacteria down. Prebiotic foods are foods that contain bacteria that support healthy populations of bacteria in our gut. Eating prebiotic foods like onions, garlic, asparagus, bananas, oats, apples, flaxseeds, and arugula help feed the beneficial gut bacteria that live in our intestines. You'll find that some of my recipes include prebiotic and probiotic foods for these reasons. You'll also see that all of these recipes are gluten-free. Research has shown that gluten damages our intestinal lining, which not only causes chronic inflammation in our gut but also contributes to poor intestinal integrity, leaving us unable to absorb essential nutrients from the food we eat. Poor intestinal integrity caused by gluten and other inflammatory foods also allows undigested food particles to move through the intestines and into the bloodstream, resulting in chronic systemic inflammation. Cruciferous vegetables like broccoli, cauliflower, radishes, and Brussels sprouts are rich in sulfur-containing compounds called glucosinolates which help our bodies eliminate waste and toxins we are exposed to. It's important to have an optimal functioning detox and elimination system to avoid overload of particles that cause inflammation throughout the body.

To be successful in following an anti-inflammatory diet, it's important to be prepared, have helpful equipment, and have the right mindset. Be prepared for the unexpected and you'll have already set yourself up for success. We all have busy lives and cooking a beautiful, nutritious meal from scratch every night may not be realistic. If this is your dilemma, it may be a good idea to cook your meals in larger batches and store leftovers in the fridge or freezer so all you need to do is warm up a delicious and nutrient-dense meal. It's also convenient to have some equipment to help you prepare a great meal with little effort and maximum nutrition. I love having my pressure cooker, slow cooker, blender, and air fryer readily available to me. These tools (and quality ingredients) allow you to make a delicious meal without compromising taste, texture, or nutrition. Finally, you have to have the right mindset. Many people fall back into eating inflammatory convenient foods after one meal where they indulge in a craving. They feel like they "blew it" and go right back to old eating habits despite all the progress they've made. Eating healthily is not black or white. It's not all or nothing. It's okay to satisfy a food craving once in a while. If you're eating a well-balanced and nutritious diet, your body is functioning at its best and on the rare occasion you decide to introduce food with less nutritional value, your body is better equipped to manage it and you're less likely to have a crazy inflammatory response than if you were eating nutrient-poor foods regularly. Even if you feel like you "blew it"–take a breath and move on, you'll have plenty of other opportunities to eat meals that are nutrient-rich and free of inflammatory triggers. You got this!

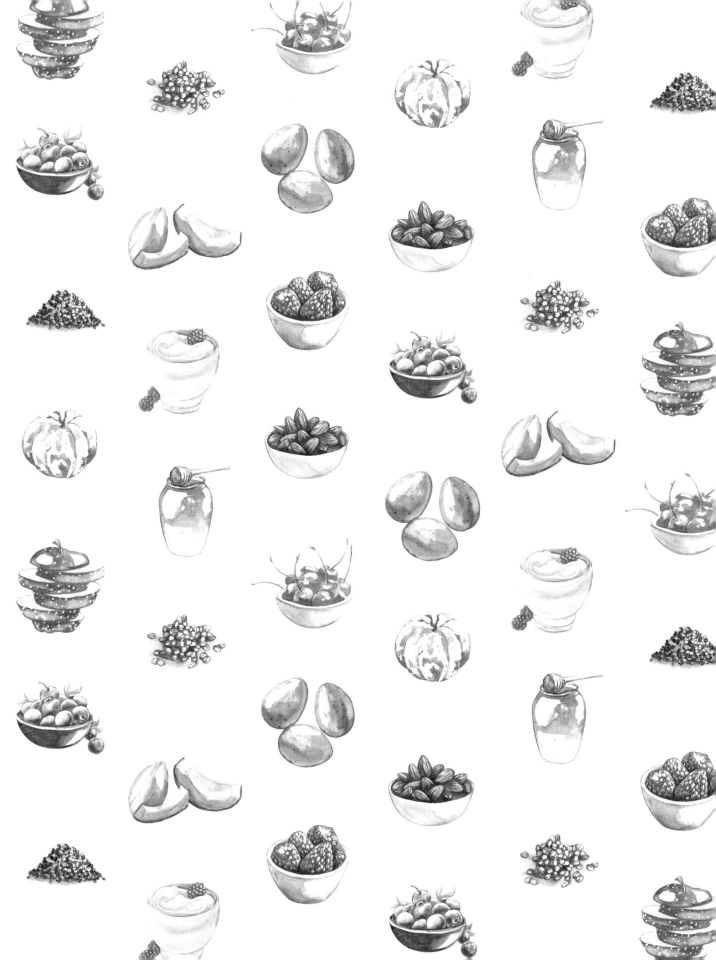

BREAKFAST

Sunday Morning Egg Bake

This dish has everything you need to enjoy a fulfilling Sunday breakfast—antioxidants, healthy fats, quality protein, and great taste! This dish can also be used for meal prep to keep your weekday breakfasts nutrient-packed while on-the-go.

INGREDIENTS

½ tablespoon avocado oil

1 lb. humanely raised breakfast sausage

10 whole pasture-raised eggs

½ teaspoon salt

¼ teaspoon black pepper

1 tablespoon nutritional yeast

½ teaspoon garlic powder

2 tablespoons milk of your choice

1 teaspoon hot sauce (optional)

1 red bell pepper, diced

1 green bell pepper, diced

½ medium onion, diced

INSTRUCTIONS

1 Preheat oven to 375°F.

2 In a 10-inch cast-iron skillet, heat the avocado oil on medium-high heat.

3 Add the sausage and cook for about 8 to 10 minutes or until golden brown.

4 While the sausage is cooking, whisk the eggs together. Add the salt, pepper, nutritional yeast, garlic powder, milk of your choice, and hot sauce. Whisk until well combined. Remove the sausage from the pan and save the fat.

5 Add the diced peppers and the onions. Sauté for about 5 to 7 minutes, or until the onions look translucent and the peppers become tender.

6 Add the sausage back to the pan with the vegetables. Sauté in the pan for 1 minute.

7 Make sure the pan is well-greased and pour the egg mixture over the sausage, peppers, and onions.

Continued...

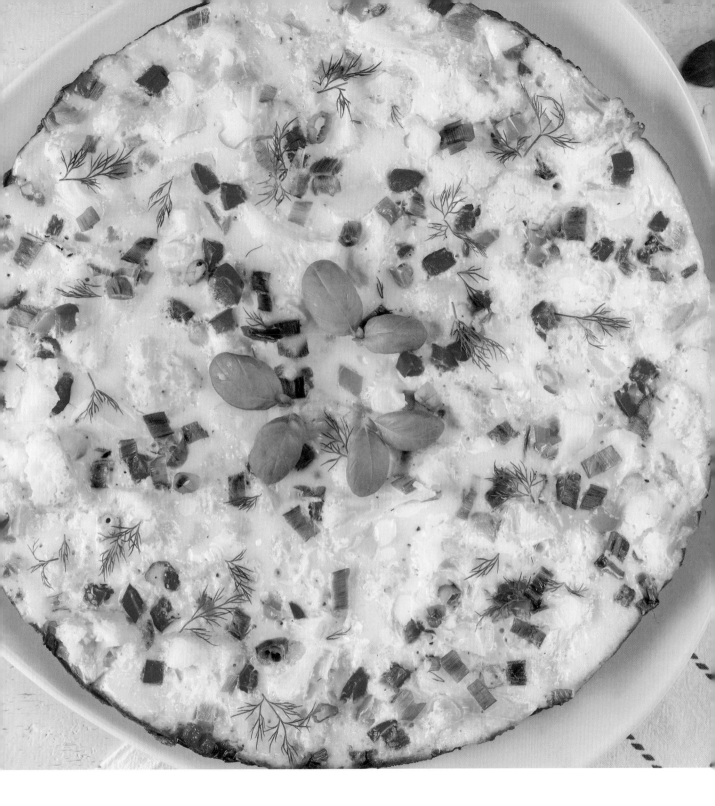

8 Let the eggs sit in the pan for about 3 minutes, then transfer to the oven.

9 Let bake for about 15 to 18 minutes or until the eggs in the center of the pan are firm.

10 Once firm, remove the pan from the oven and let sit for a few minutes.

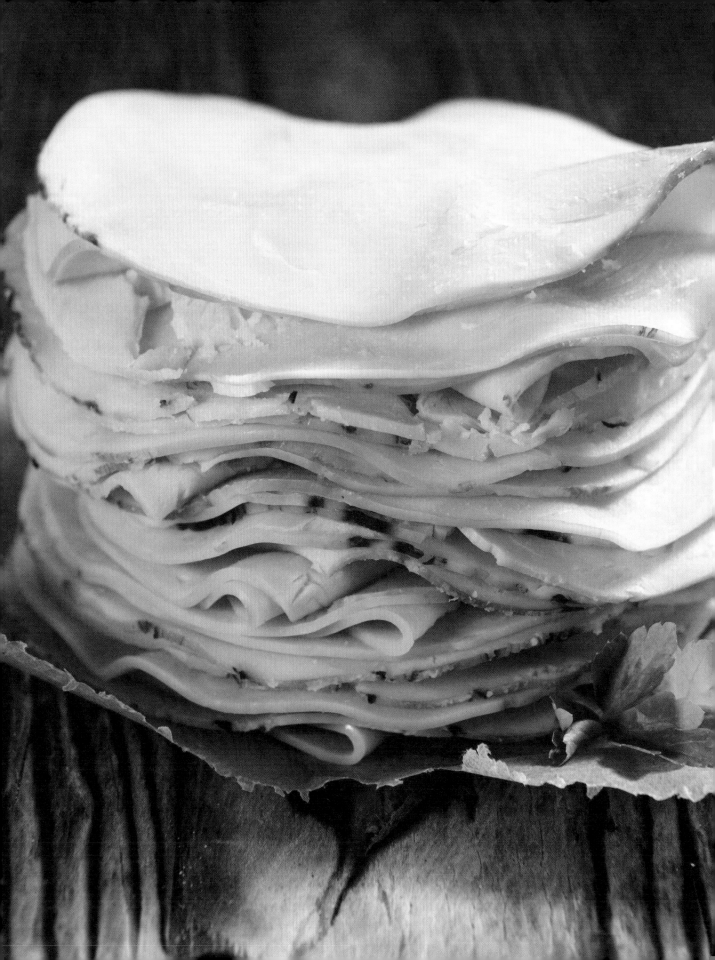

Lean Breakfast Wrap

This breakfast wrap is a little different in that it uses sliced turkey as the tortilla. It's a delicious recipe that helps you avoid the inflammatory immune reactions associated with gluten. This wrap is a quick and easy breakfast that is high in quality protein but guaranteed to keep you full and fueled throughout the day. Best of all, this wrap is rich in anti-inflammatory nutrients like choline, vitamin A, vitamin C, vitamin K, omega-3 fatty acids, potassium, and B vitamins.

INGREDIENTS

2 large whole pasture-raised eggs

Pinch or ⅛ teaspoon sea salt

Pinch or ⅛ teaspoon black pepper

Coconut oil cooking spray

1 cup baby kale, chopped

2 oz. sliced organic turkey

¼ Hass avocado, cut into thin slices

INSTRUCTIONS

1 In a small bowl, whisk eggs together and season with salt and pepper.

2 Coat a small skillet with cooking spray. Heat the skillet over medium heat. Add chopped baby kale and sauté for about 3 minutes.

3 Add the eggs to the skillet and cook until the eggs are at the desired consistency (about 6 minutes for soft scrambled eggs, about 8 minutes for firm eggs).

4 Remove the eggs from the pan, then place the turkey slices on the skillet to warm for about 1 minute. Transfer the turkey slices from the pan onto a plate, place the eggs on the turkey slices, and top with avocado.

5 Feel free to garnish with fresh herbs of your choice, then fold the turkey slices or roll it into a wrap.

Overnight Oats

Oats are an excellent anti-inflammatory food due to their many gut health benefits. A healthy gut means a healthy immune system that reduces systemic inflammation. The oats act as a prebiotic, which means that they support healthy gut bacteria populations. This recipe provides the necessary fat, fiber, and protein you need to stabilize your blood sugar and get you ready for the day.

INGREDIENTS

⅔ cup unsweetened vanilla almond milk

1 scoop grass-fed collagen peptides

½ cup gluten-free rolled oats

½ tablespoon chia seeds

½ tablespoon hemp seeds

⅓ cup chopped strawberries

¼ cup blueberries

2 tablespoons organic maple syrup (optional)

½ teaspoon cinnamon

¼ teaspoon allspice

INSTRUCTIONS

1 In a small bowl, add the milk and collagen peptides and whisk well.

2 Add all of the ingredients to a mason jar or desired container. Stir well or close the container and shake well to mix.

3 Place the oat container into the fridge overnight.

4 Heat the oats in the morning and add extra cinnamon before serving.

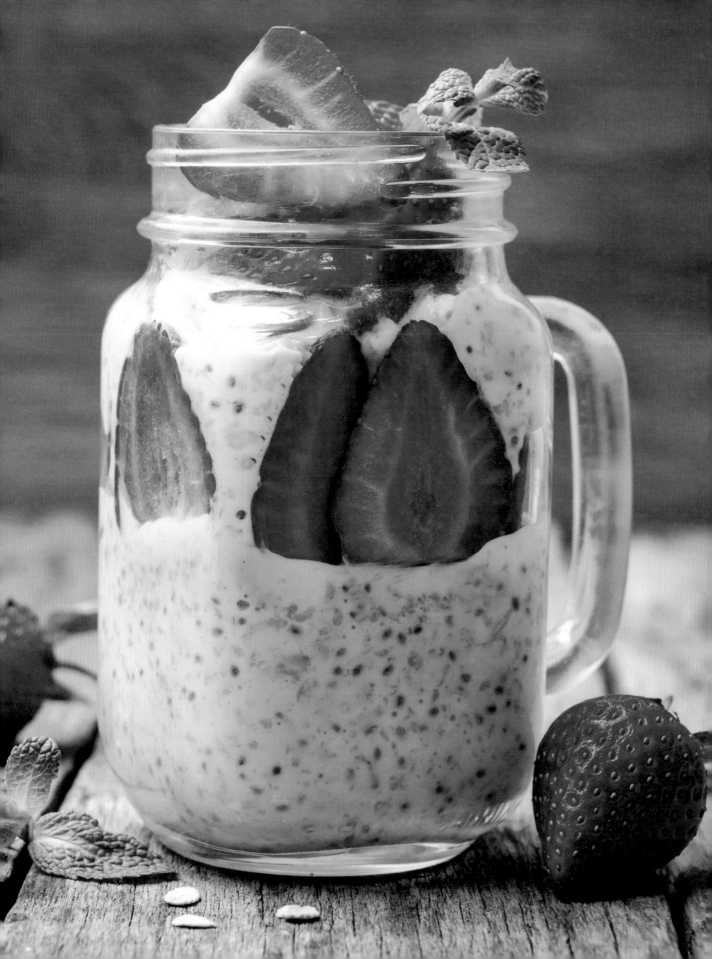

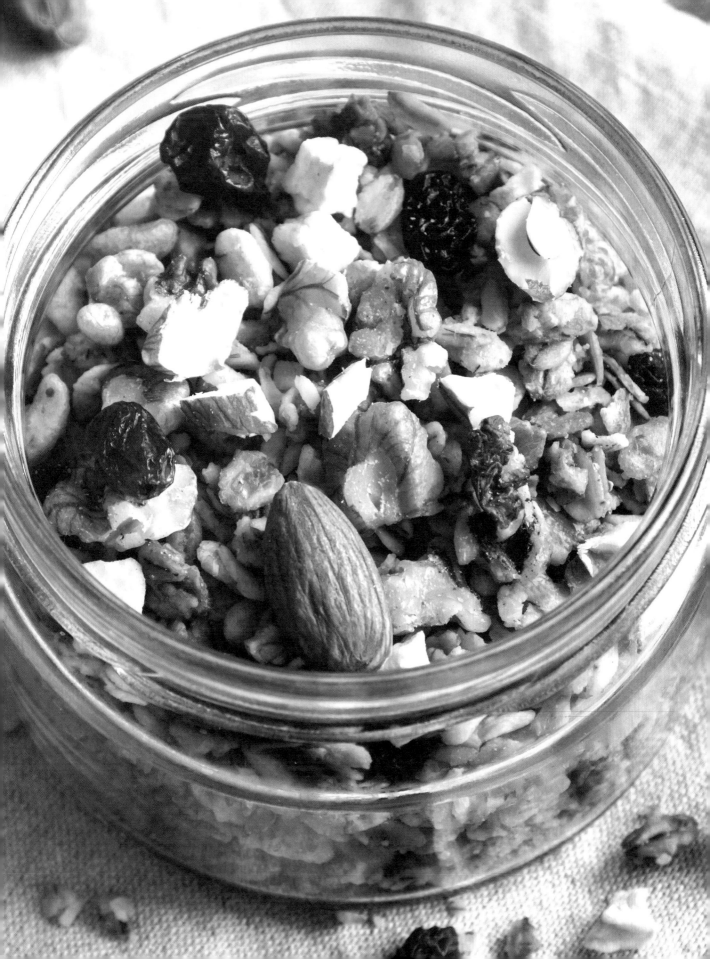

Homemade Granola

Ditch the store-bought granola. This homemade granola is packed with anti-inflammatory ingredients like omega-3 fatty acids, antioxidants, and polyphenols. This recipe helps reduce the inflammation in our bodies associated with heart disease, obesity, and cancer risk.

INGREDIENTS

1 cup almonds

1 cup pecan pieces

1 cup hazelnuts, chopped

1 cup shredded coconut, unsweetened

⅓ cup pumpkin seeds

1 tablespoon chia seeds

1 tablespoon flaxseed meal

¼ cup almond butter

¼ cup maple syrup

1 teaspoon vanilla extract

¼ teaspoon nutmeg

¼ teaspoon cinnamon

1 cup dried cherries, unsweetened

INSTRUCTIONS

1 Preheat oven to 325°F and line baking sheet with parchment paper.

2 In a food processor, add the almonds, pecans, hazelnuts, coconut, pumpkin seeds, chia seeds, flaxseed meal, almond butter, maple syrup, vanilla, nutmeg, and cinnamon.

3 Pulse until the ingredients are well mixed and begin to clump together. Do not overmix.

4 Place the crumble on a prepared baking sheet and spread the mixture out.

5 Place the baking sheet in the oven for about 20 minutes, stirring the crumble every 5 minutes.

6 Remove the baking sheet from the oven and let the granola cool completely.

7 Mix in the cherries and enjoy either plain, with yogurt (if you can tolerate dairy), or with a chia seed pudding (see recipe on page 20).

Overnight Very Berry Chia Seed Pudding

This chia seed pudding is a delicious alternative to yogurt or pudding because it cuts out the abundance of sugar that creates inflammation within our bodies. Luckily, chia seeds are also rich in fiber, anti-inflammatory omega 3-fatty acids, and the antioxidants and polyphenols that come with berries. This pudding is a great alternative for those who do not tolerate dairy well.

INGREDIENTS

1 can full-fat coconut milk

⅔ cup water or your favorite dairy-free milk (I like to use oat milk or almond milk)

⅓ cup frozen blueberries

⅓ cup frozen raspberries

⅓ cup frozen strawberries

3 scoops grass-fed collagen peptides

1 tablespoon raw honey

1 teaspoon vanilla extract

⅓ cup chia seeds

INSTRUCTIONS

1 Add the coconut milk, water or milk, berries, collagen peptides, honey, and vanilla to a blender and blend until the mixture is very smooth.

2 Transfer the mixture to a large bowl or Tupperware. With a whisk, slowly add in the chia seeds.

3 Continue whisking for an extra 2 minutes, then transfer the mixture into individual mason jars or airtight containers.

4 Chill the pudding in the fridge overnight and serve the next morning for breakfast with granola and extra fresh berries.

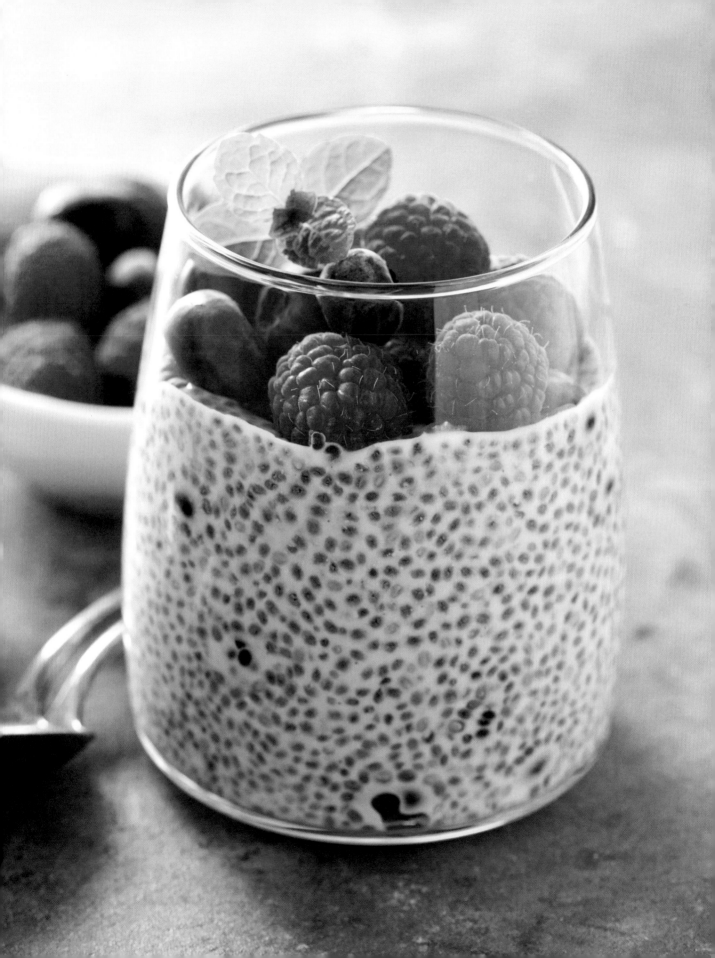

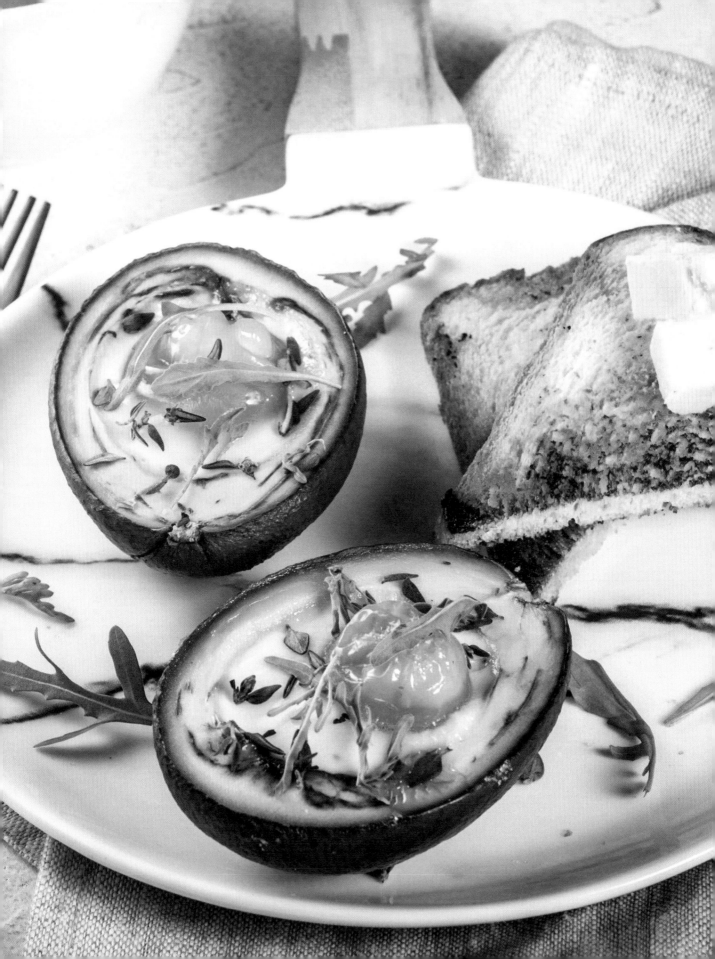

Avocado Egg Cups

These egg cups are the perfect on-the-go breakfast and are packed with high-quality fat and protein. Not to mention avocado and pasture-raised eggs are rich in omega-3 fatty acids, choline, potassium, B vitamins, and other antioxidants that support your immune system when inflammatory triggers try to sneak in.

INGREDIENTS

2 large Hass avocados

2 oz. your choice of cooked chopped bacon or sausage, cooked vegetables, or smoked salmon

4 whole pasture-raised eggs

Pinch or ⅛ teaspoon sea salt

Pinch or ⅛ teaspoon black pepper

½ tablespoon chives or parsley (fresh or dried)

Pinch or ⅛ teaspoon crushed red pepper (optional)

INSTRUCTIONS

1 Heat oven to 425°F.

2 Cut the avocados in half and remove the pits. Scoop out some flesh just a bit larger than the size of the pit in order to create a bigger well.

3 Place the avocados faceup in a small baking dish (or slice a thin layer off of the back of the avocado to keep them from tipping over).

4 Fill the cavities of the avocados with cooked vegetables or protein of your choice.

5 Crack one egg into each avocado cavity. If needed, remove some of the egg white before baking to avoid spilling over.

6 Season with salt and pepper.

7 Bake for about 15 minutes, or until the eggs are cooked to your liking.

8 Garnish with fresh herbs and crushed red pepper, if using.

Veggie Egg Muffin Cups

These muffins are a delicious and fun way to enjoy eggs in the morning or are a great option if you're looking to meal prep for weekday breakfasts. The mushrooms are the star in this recipe due to their many anti-inflammatory compounds like polysaccharides, terpenes, and other phenolic compounds that support our immune system and combat inflammatory triggers.

INGREDIENTS

2 tablespoons avocado oil

¾ cup red bell pepper, chopped

¾ cup green bell pepper, chopped

¾ cup cremini mushrooms, chopped

½ cup yellow onion, unsweetened

2 cups baby spinach, chopped

12 whole pasture-raised eggs

2 tablespoons almond milk

1 tablespoon nutritional yeast

Continued...

INSTRUCTIONS

1 Preheat the oven to 350°F.

2 In a cast-iron skillet, heat the avocado oil on medium-high heat and add the peppers, mushrooms, and onions. Sauté for about 7 to 8 minutes.

3 Add the spinach to the pan and sauté for another 3 to 5 minutes. Remove all of the vegetables from the pan.

4 Crack the eggs in a large mixing bowl. Add the almond milk, nutritional yeast, spices, and hot sauce and scramble until the mix is well combined.

5 Spray a 12-cup muffin pan with cooking spray. Spoon the vegetables into each muffin cup. Carefully pour the eggs over each vegetable cup. Place the pan into the oven and cook the egg muffins for about 25 to 28 minutes.

6 Remove the pan from the oven, let cool, and serve.

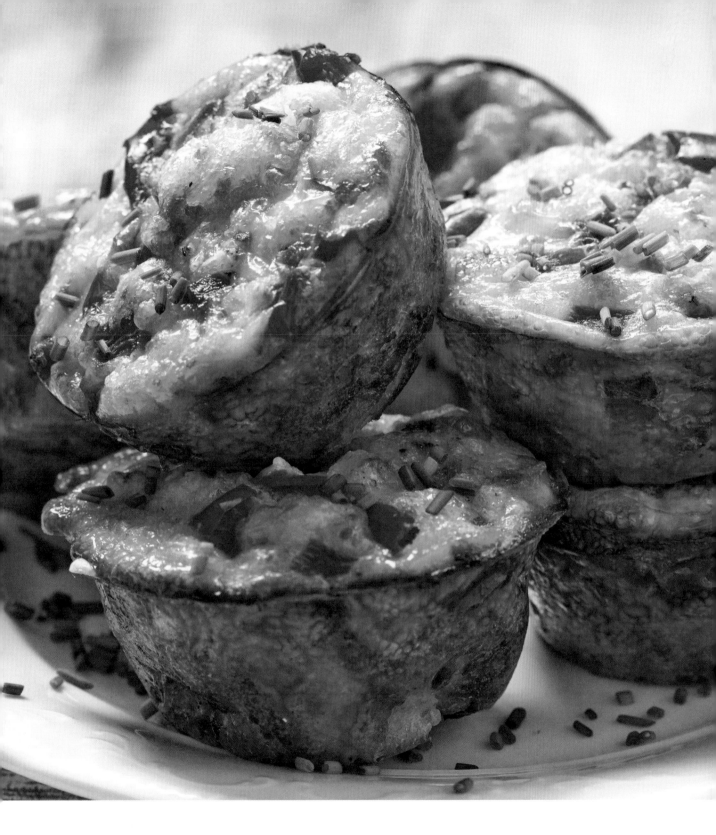

| 1 tablespoon chives | ½ teaspoon salt | ½ teaspoon hot sauce |
| 1 teaspoon garlic powder | ½ teaspoon black pepper | Cooking spray |

Sweet Potato Breakfast Skillet

Sweet potatoes are high in beta-carotene that helps your body defend itself from inflammatory triggers. Kale is also packed with antioxidants, including beta-carotene, vitamin C, and quercetin that help protect your body from damage caused by inflammation.

INGREDIENTS

6 strips humanely raised bacon, chopped into thick pieces

1 medium red onion, diced

2 garlic cloves, minced

1 red bell pepper, diced

1 large sweet potato, peeled and diced into small cubes

Salt, to taste, plus ½ teaspoon

Black pepper, to taste, plus ¼ teaspoon

2 tablespoons water

2 cups kale leaves, stems removed, roughly chopped

½ tablespoon nutritional yeast

Continued...

INSTRUCTIONS

1   Heat a large cast-iron skillet over medium heat. Add the bacon and sauté until golden and crispy. Remove the bacon pieces and leave the fat.

2   Add the diced onion, garlic, and red bell pepper to the pan. Sauté for about 3 minutes or until onions become aromatic.

3   Add the diced sweet potato to the pan. Cook the sweet potato for about 12 to 15 minutes, stirring often. Add a pinch of salt and pepper. Add the water and place a lid over the mixture for about 3 to 5 minutes or until the sweet potatoes are fork-tender.

4   Return the bacon to the pan, add the kale, spices, ½ teaspoon salt, and ¼ teaspoon pepper and stir for an additional 4 minutes or until the kale begins to wilt.

5   Use a spatula to create 4 wells in the hash. Spray each well lightly with cooking spray, if needed. Crack an egg into each well and cook until the eggs are done to your liking.

6   Garnish with chives and serve.

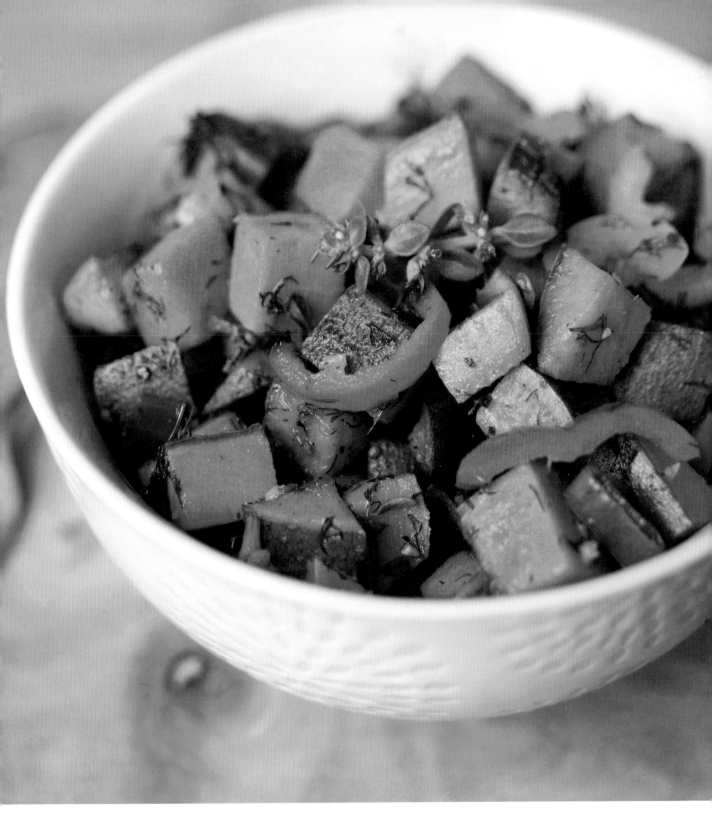

| ½ teaspoon cumin | ¼ teaspoon paprika | 4 whole pasture-raised eggs |
| 1 teaspoon garlic powder | Cooking spray | ¼ cup chives, diced, for garnish |

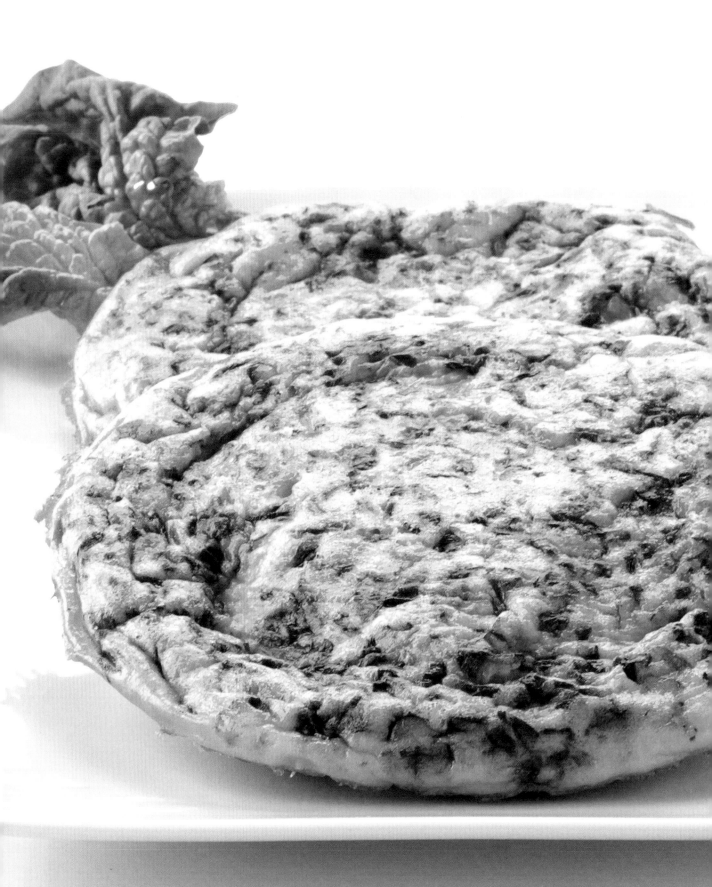

Green Eggs

Eggs are packed with vitamin A, choline, vitamin B12, calcium, zinc, vitamin D, selenium, and much more. All of these nutrients support your immune system's ability to ward off inflammation and increase your body's natural ability to detox waste. The quality fat and protein also help you feel fueled and energized throughout your morning.

INGREDIENTS

4 whole pasture-raised eggs

2 tablespoons non-dairy milk

1 teaspoon nutritional yeast

Cooking spray

4 cup spinach, chopped

¼ cup red onion, chopped

¼ cup green bell pepper, diced

½ teaspoon onion powder

Sea salt and black pepper, to taste

3 tablespoons grass-fed butter or ghee

INSTRUCTIONS

1 In a medium bowl, scramble the eggs with non-dairy milk and nutritional yeast.

2 Heat a medium skillet on the stove and coat with cooking spray. Add the spinach, onion, and pepper and sauté for about 5 to 7 minutes. Season with onion powder and add salt and pepper to taste.

3 Add the butter and stir in the vegetables until the butter is melted.

4 Add the scrambled eggs and cook for 6 minutes or until desired doneness is reached.

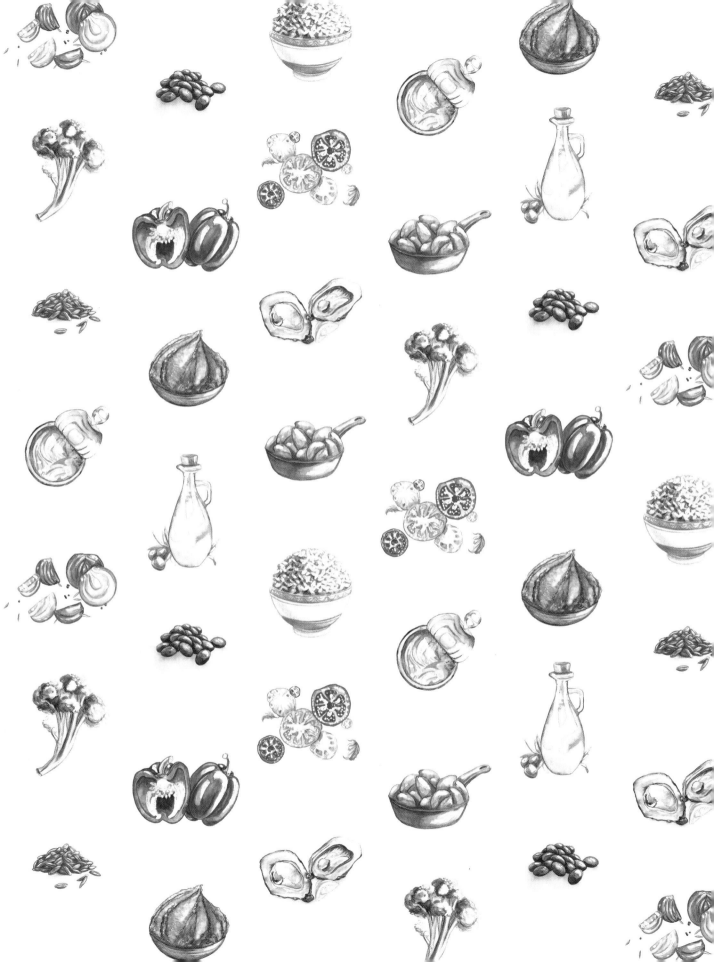

SNACKS & SIDES

Krissy's Crispy Chickpeas

The protein and fiber content makes these a great snack, but they're also a great substitute for salad croutons. Croutons are made with lots of pro-inflammatory ingredients that contribute to many chronic health issues. These crispy chickpeas add the perfect crunch to your salad without all the ugly health consequences. Chickpeas are pretty versatile, so you can simply season them with salt or add your favorite seasonings to elevate the flavor of your salad.

INGREDIENTS

1 can (15 oz.) chickpeas, rinsed and drained

1 tablespoon avocado oil

1 tablespoon nutritional yeast

1 tablespoon garlic powder

½ teaspoon onion powder

¼ teaspoon chili powder

½ teaspoon sea salt

Pinch of black pepper

INSTRUCTIONS

1 Preheat the air fryer to 400°F.

2 Dry the chickpeas very well with paper towels. They should be completely dry.

3 Add all of the ingredients into a bowl and toss well. Pour the ingredients into the air fryer basket.

4 Cook for about 10 to 12 minutes. Shake basket halfway through.

5 Once finished cooking, remove the chickpeas from the basket and let them cool on a plate.

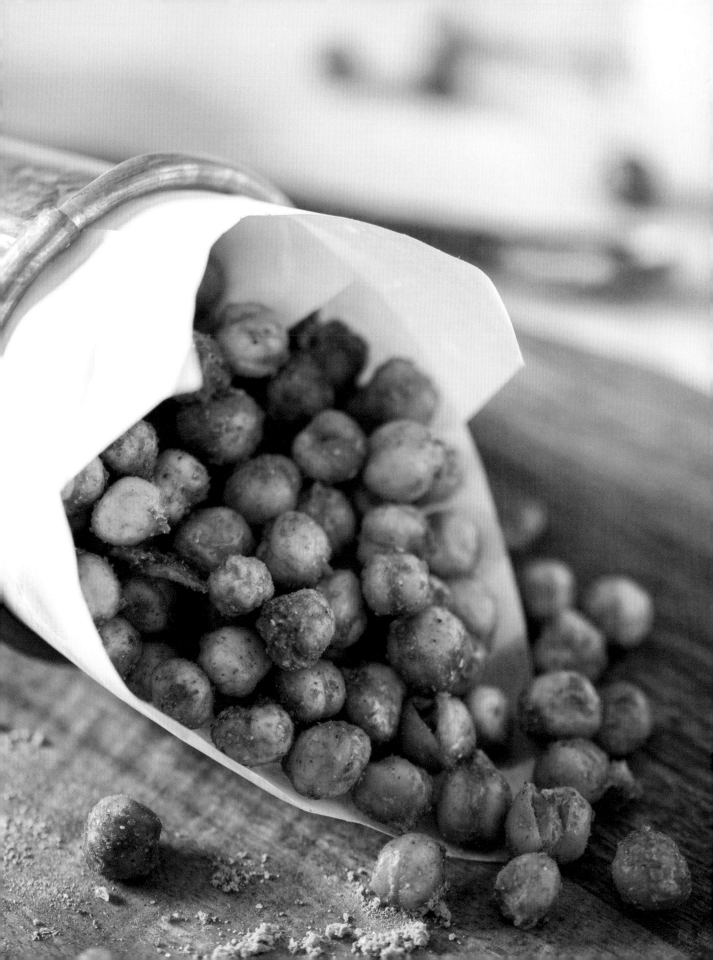

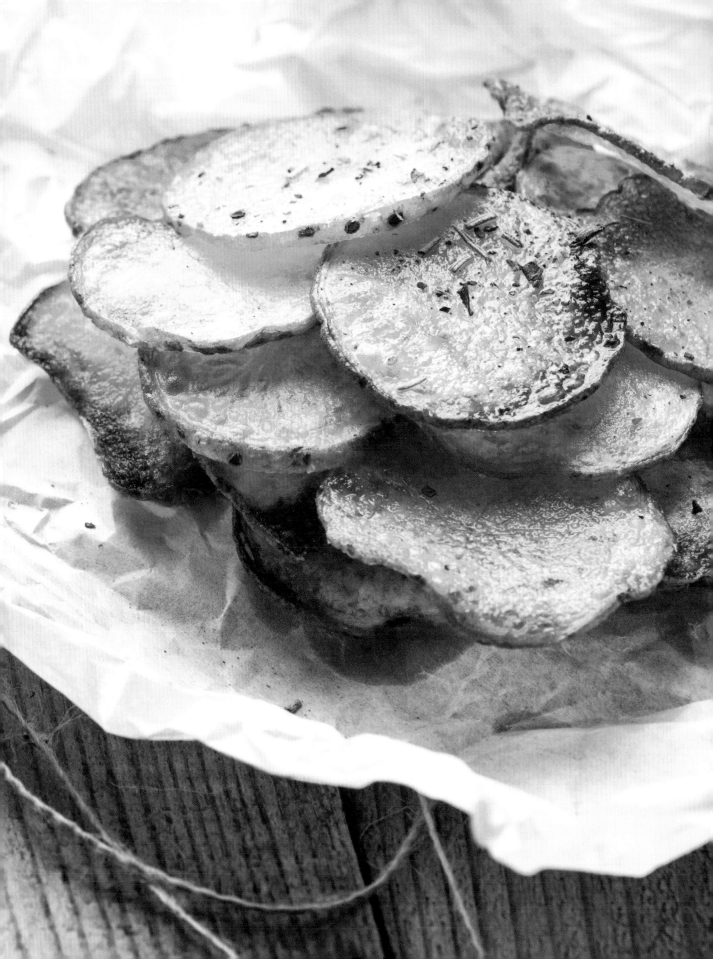

Savory Potato Chips

These potatoes are a great substitute for potato chips or french fries. The recipe avoids inflammatory oils and seasonings and instead calls for olive oil, which is high in anti-inflammatory omega-3 fatty acids.

INGREDIENTS

4-6 medium red skin or Yukon gold potatoes, sliced about ¼ inch thick

3 tablespoons olive oil

1 tablespoon minced garlic

1 teaspoon Italian seasoning

½ teaspoon garlic powder

½ teaspoon salt

¼ teaspoon black pepper

INSTRUCTIONS

1 Preheat the oven to 400°F.

2 In a medium mixing bowl, combine all of the ingredients and toss well to coat. Lay each potato slice on a baking sheet in a single layer. Do not overlap the potatoes.

3 Place the baking sheet in the oven and bake for about 30 to 40 minutes or until potatoes become deep golden brown and crispy.

Pumpkin Spice Pecans

These pecans make the perfect snack. Pecans also contain fat-soluble vitamins and essential minerals that support your health and help prevent chronic diseases.

INGREDIENTS

3 cups pecan halves

⅓ cup maple syrup

2 teaspoons pumpkin pie spice

INSTRUCTIONS

1 Preheat oven to 350°F.

2 In a large mixing bowl, combine the pecans, maple syrup, and pumpkin pie spice. Toss well to combine.

3 Place all of the nuts on a sheet pan lined with parchment paper. Place the pan in the oven for about 10 minutes, checking on the pecans at the halfway point and stirring occasionally.

4 Take the pan out of the oven and let the pecans cool before handling.

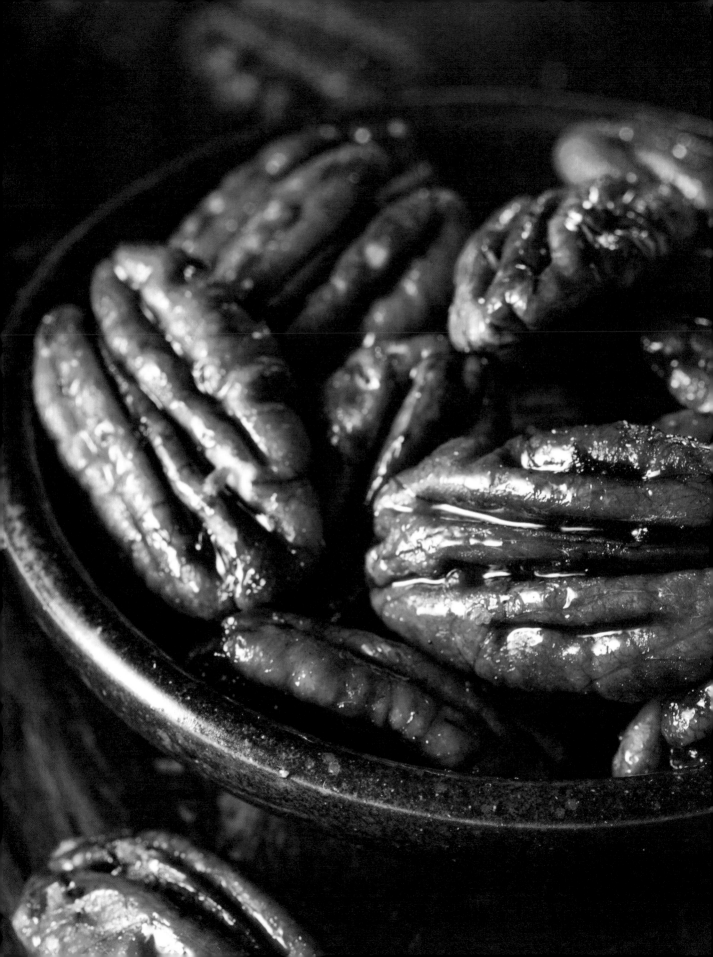

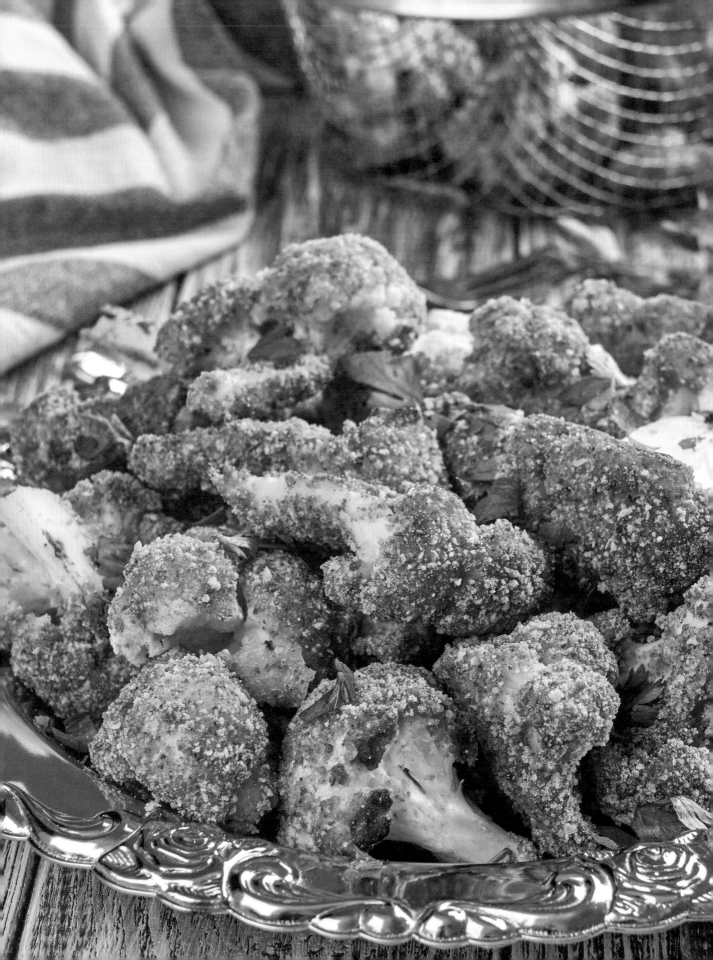

"Cheesy" Cauli Bites

This is a great side dish to add to any meal. Nutritional yeast is a great substitute for cheese when trying to avoid inflammation associated with dairy intake. Cauliflower is also a great vegetable to support your immune system and liver detox.

INGREDIENTS

1 small cauliflower head, cut into florets

2 tablespoons olive oil

2 tablespoons nutritional yeast

1 teaspoon garlic powder

¼ teaspoon smoked paprika

½ teaspoon salt

Cooking spray

INSTRUCTIONS

1   In a large bowl, combine the cauliflower florets with olive oil and the seasonings. Toss well with a spoon or tongs.

2   Spray the air fryer basket with cooking spray. Place the cauliflower in the basket and spray the tops with cooking spray.

3   Cook at 400°F for about 10 to 15 minutes. Be sure to stop and toss cauliflower at the halfway point.

Buffalo Cauliflower

Another creative and tasty way to use cauliflower. These bad boys can be eaten alone or even tossed into a green chicken salad for extra heat. Cayenne pepper (found here in the Frank's Red Hot) contains capsaicin. Capsaicin has been shown to help reduce pain associated with inflammation.

INGREDIENTS

1-2 whole pasture-raised eggs

1 cup almond flour

½ teaspoon sea salt

2 teaspoons garlic powder

1 large head cauliflower, cut into florets

1 cup Frank's Red Hot Sauce

1 teaspoon coconut aminos

INSTRUCTIONS

1 Preheat oven to 425°F.

2 In a shallow bowl, whisk the eggs very well. In a separate bowl, combine the almond flour, salt, and garlic powder.

3 Dip each floret in the eggs and then coat the florets in the flour mixture.

4 Place the florets on the baking sheet and then place the pan in the oven for about 25 minutes, or until cauliflower is golden brown.

5 While the cauliflower is baking, whisk the hot sauce and aminos.

6 Remove the cauliflower from the oven and let the florets cool for about 10 minutes.

7 Pour the hot sauce over the cauliflower and toss to combine with tongs.

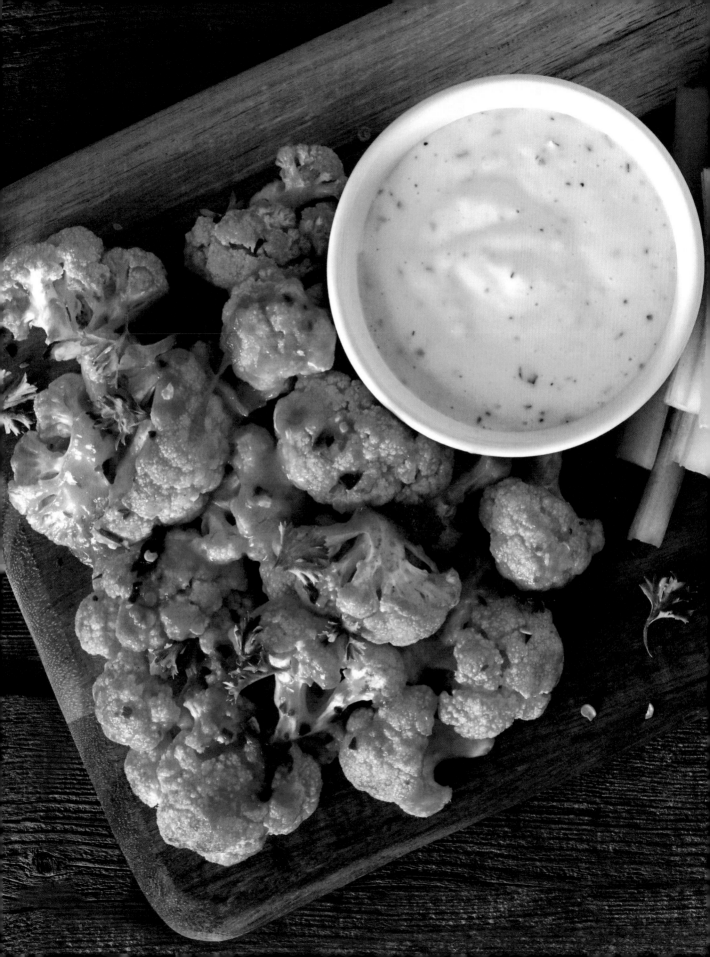

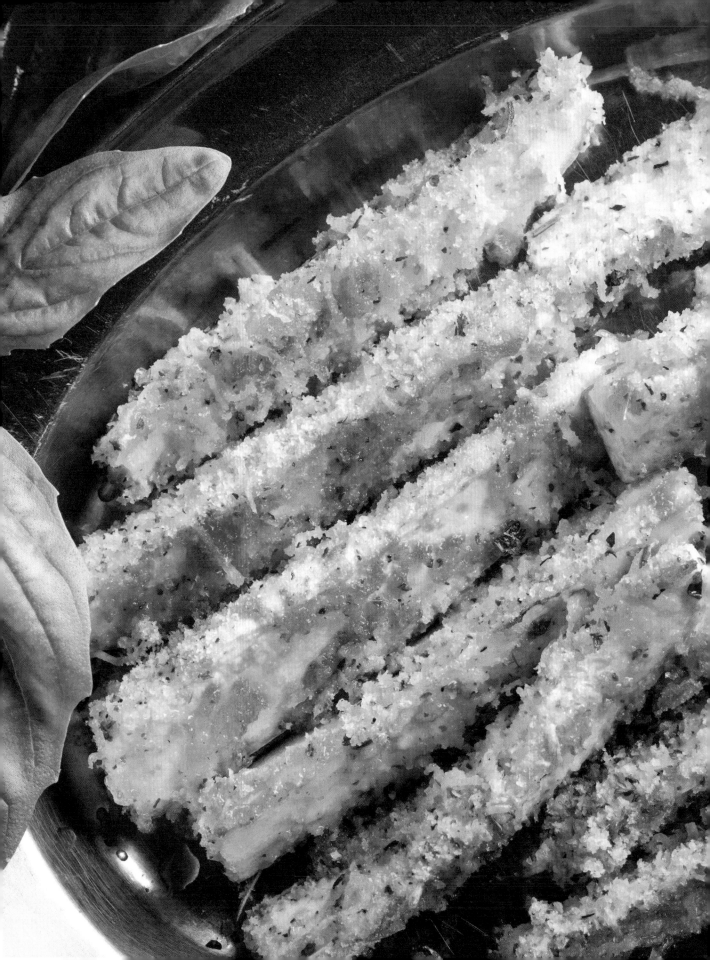

Zucchini Fries

French fries will always hold a special place in my heart and sometimes I need something to bring me a little comfort without straying away from the foods that will serve my health. These zucchini fries have a great crunch and pair well with your favorite dipping sauce. Did I mention that zucchini is rich in antioxidants? Lutein and zeaxanthin in zucchini keep your immune system strong against inflammatory triggers.

INGREDIENTS

2 whole pasture-raised eggs, beaten very well

1 cup almond meal

1 tablespoon nutritional yeast

½ teaspoon salt

1 teaspoon garlic powder

1 teaspoon onion powder

2 large zucchinis, cut lengthwise into quarters

INSTRUCTIONS

1 Preheat air fryer to 400°F.

2 In a small bowl, beat the eggs very well. In a separate bowl, combine the almond meal, nutritional yeast, salt, garlic powder, and onion powder.

3 Working with 1 piece at a time, dip each zucchini piece into the eggs and then place each one in the almond meal mixture, coating well.

4 Place the zucchini in a single layer in the fryer basket. Cook for about 15 to 20 minutes in the air fryer or until the zucchini becomes golden brown. Remove the zucchini fries and let cool.

Bacon Wrapped Zucchini Fries

This simple veggie dish is a great snack or a delicious side dish to any meal.

INGREDIENTS

4 medium zucchinis, cut in half and then lengthwise

12-16 strips humanely raised bacon

Pinch of allspice (optional)

INSTRUCTIONS

1 Preheat the oven to 400°F.

2 Wrap each zucchini fry with a slice of bacon and place the fry on a baking sheet.

3 Place the baking sheet in the oven and cook for about 30 minutes or until the bacon becomes crispy.

4 Remove from oven and garnish with a pinch of allspice, if desired.

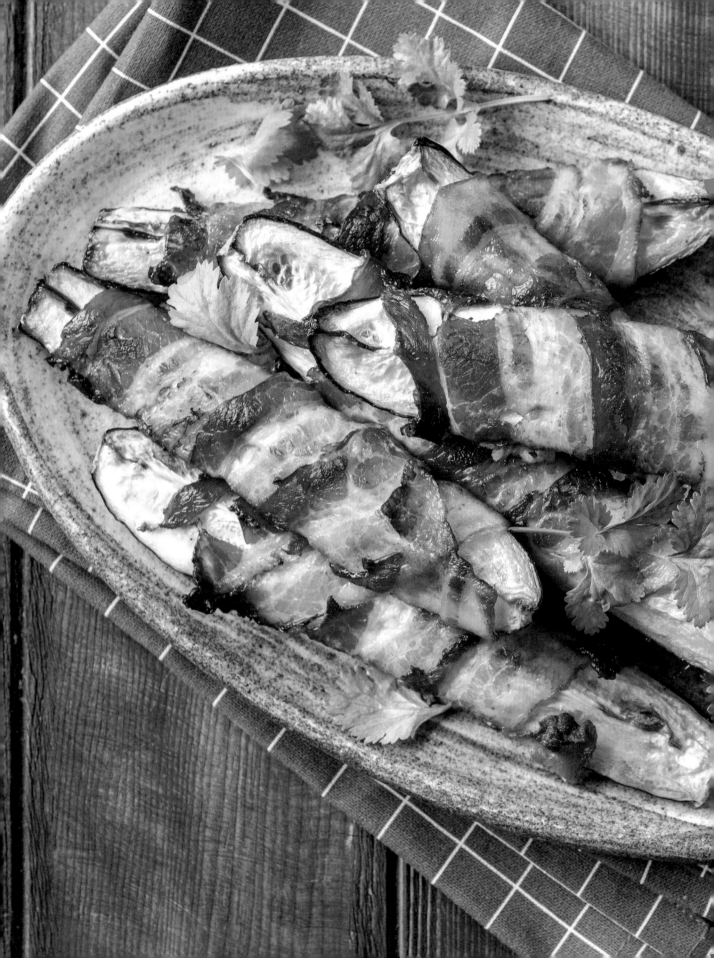

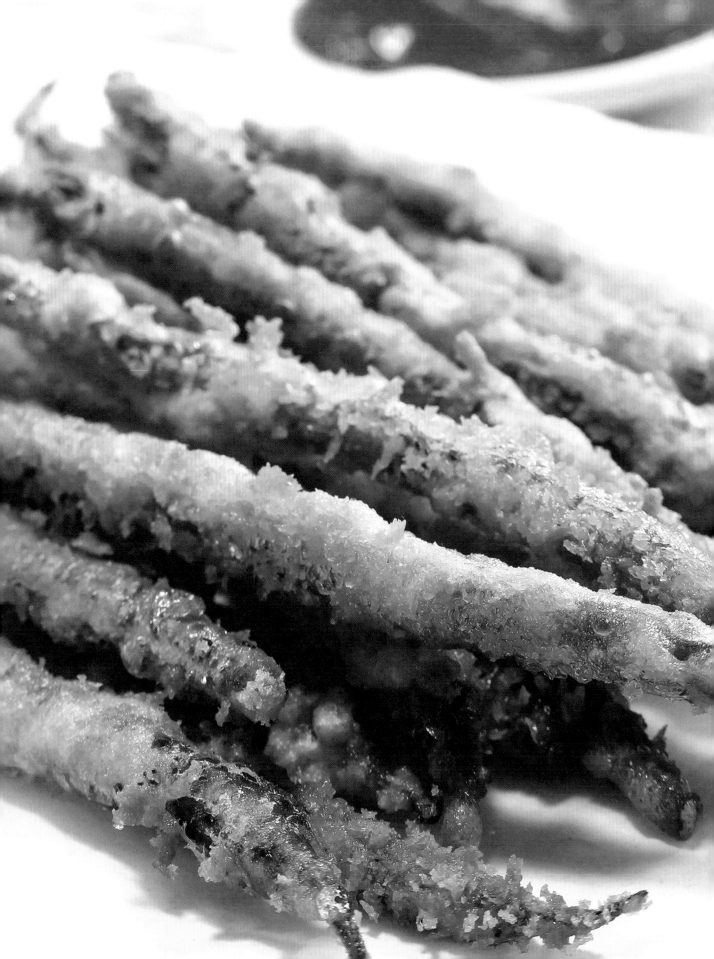

Air Fryer Garlic Green Beans

This side dish has tons of fiber which will keep you full and satisfied.
Pair it with your favorite protein for a perfect meal.

INGREDIENTS

1 lb. fresh green beans (trimmed)

2 tablespoons olive oil

1 teaspoon garlic powder

4 cloves garlic, minced

¼ teaspoon lemon zest

Salt and pepper, to taste

¼ cup sliced roasted almonds (optional)

INSTRUCTIONS

1 Preheat the air fryer to 370°F.

2 In a mixing bowl, toss the green beans with olive oil, garlic powder, minced garlic, lemon zest, and salt and pepper to taste.

3 Cook the green beans in the air fryer for about 7 to 10 minutes. When halfway cooked, toss the beans in the basket.

4 Remove the green beans from the air fryer basket and top with sliced almonds, if desired.

Gluten-Free Italian Pasta Salad

Perfect for a summertime BBQ, this recipe allows you to make a homemade dressing without all the added sugars and inflammatory hydrogenated oils of a store-bought dressing.

INGREDIENTS

Salad

8 oz. gluten-free pasta of choice (I like to use Fusilli pasta)

⅓ cup roasted red peppers from a jar, thinly sliced

1 medium green bell pepper, diced

1 pint cherry tomatoes, halved

½ medium red onion, thinly sliced or diced

3 medium carrots, diced

2 celery stalks, diced

⅓ cup sun-dried tomatoes, chopped

⅓ cup fresh parsley, chopped

6 oz. fresh mozzarella, cubed (optional, omit for a dairy-free version)

Continued...

INSTRUCTIONS

1 Cook the pasta according to the instructions. Run cold water through the pasta and set aside.

2 Prepare the contents of the salad and place them into a large bowl.

3 In a small bowl, whisk the dressing ingredients together.

4 Add the cooked and cooled pasta into the salad bowl along with the dressing. Combine well.

5 Let the salad sit for about 30 minutes in the fridge before serving.

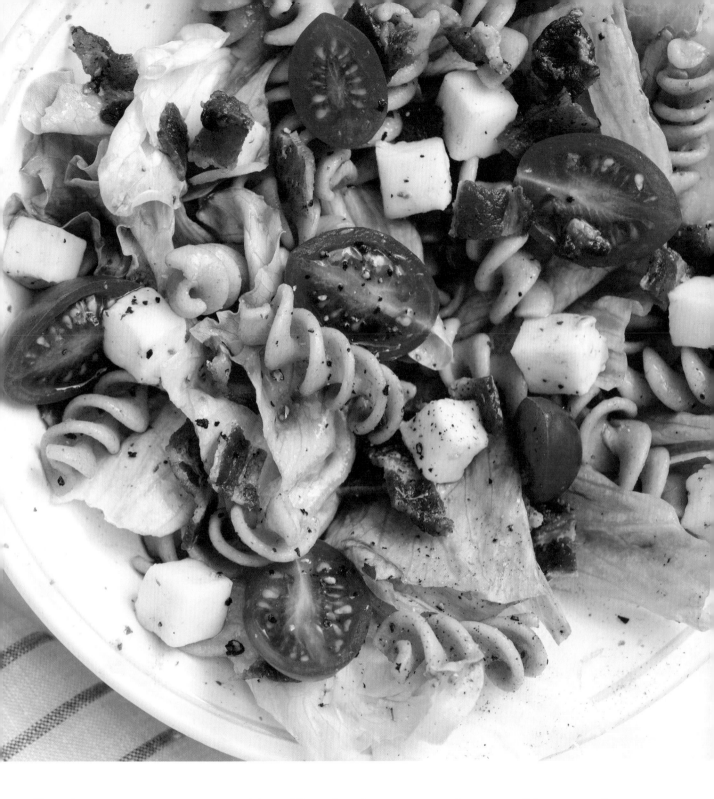

Dressing

½ cup olive oil

3 tablespoons apple cider vinegar or red wine vinegar

Juice of ½ medium lemon

1-2 garlic cloves, minced

2 teaspoons Italian seasoning

1 teaspoon Dijon mustard

½ teaspoon salt

¼ teaspoon black pepper

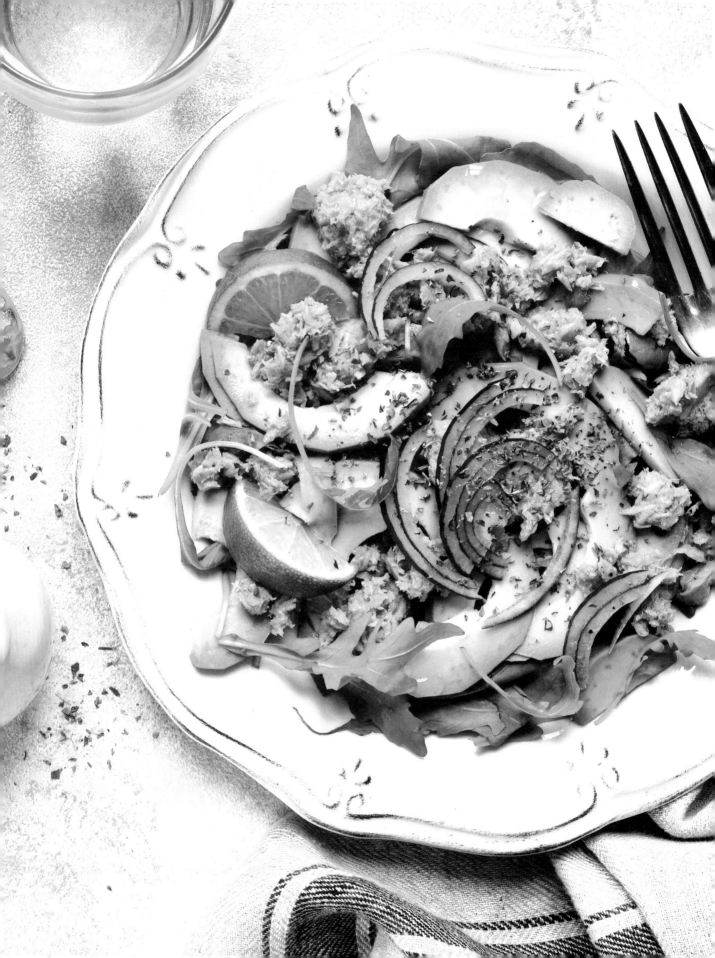

Avocado Tuna Salad

This is a great alternative to tuna salad. Instead of mayo, the recipe calls for avocado, which provides more immune-boosting nutrients and anti-inflammatory fatty acids.

INGREDIENTS

1 medium avocado, smashed

Juice of ½ lemon

2 tablespoons diced celery

2 tablespoons chopped red onion

1 (5 oz.) can albacore tuna, drained

¼ teaspoon garlic powder

Sea salt and black pepper, to taste

INSTRUCTIONS

1 Mash the avocado in a shallow bowl and add the lemon juice, celery, and onion. Mix well.

2 Add the drained tuna, garlic powder, sea salt, and pepper.

3 Mix well and serve on top of a salad or gluten-free or sprouted grain bread.

Tomato & Cucumber Greek Salad

Rich in anti-inflammatory omega-3 fatty acids, this simple and tasty salad is designed to support your health goals.

INGREDIENTS

3 cups English hothouse cucumbers, coarsely chopped

1 large tomato, coarsely chopped

1 green bell pepper, coarsely chopped

½ medium red onion, thinly sliced

½ cup Kalamata olives, pitted and halved

3 tablespoons extra-virgin olive oil

1½ tablespoons red wine vinegar

Juice of ½ small lemon

½ teaspoon sea salt

¼ teaspoon black pepper

1 tablespoon dried oregano

¼ cup coarsely chopped fresh parsley (optional)

4 oz. package feta, crumbled (optional, omit if sensitive to dairy)

INSTRUCTIONS

1 Prepare all the vegetables and olives and place them into a medium-sized bowl.

2 In a small bowl, whisk the olive oil, red wine vinegar, lemon juice, salt, pepper, and oregano to make a vinaigrette.

3 Add the vinaigrette to the bowl and toss to combine.

4 Add the parsley and feta cheese, if desired, and serve.

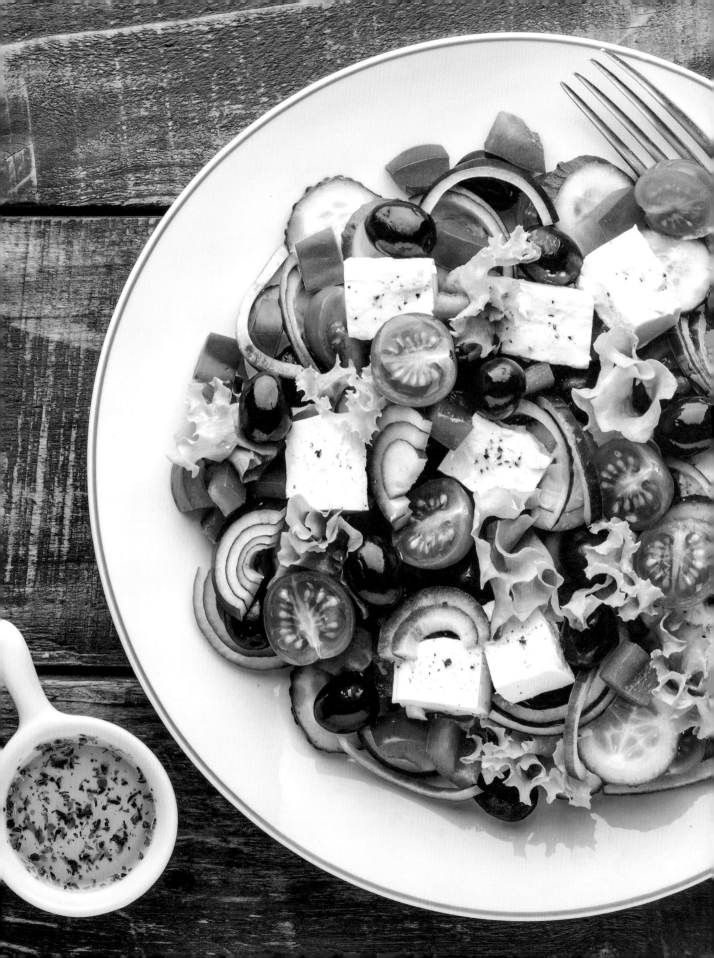

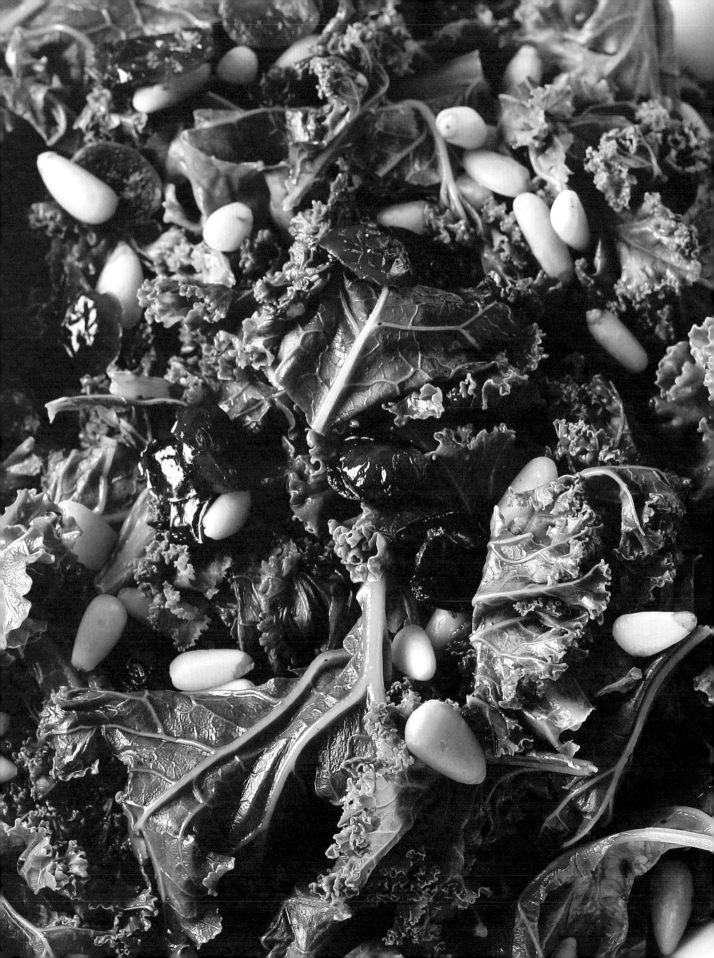

Fall Kale Salad

This nutrient-packed salad has everything you need to combat inflammation:
fiber, antioxidants, polyphenols, probiotics, and prebiotics.

INGREDIENTS

1 large bunch of curly green or red kale, washed and patted dry, tough stems removed, chopped or torn by hand into bite-size pieces

¼ teaspoon sea salt

3 tablespoons extra-virgin olive oil

2 tablespoons apple cider vinegar

¼ teaspoon black pepper

1 medium apple, sliced thin

1 small onion, sliced thin

1 medium carrot, sliced thin

¼ cup dried cranberries

3 tablespoons roasted pumpkin seeds

⅓ cup roasted walnuts, chopped

INSTRUCTIONS

1 Place the chopped kale into a large bowl.

2 Sprinkle with sea salt and a tablespoon olive oil.

3 Massage the kale until the leaves start to soften, about 10 minutes.

4 Whisk the remaining olive oil, apple cider vinegar, and pepper in a small bowl and set aside.

5 Toss the remaining ingredients with the kale.

6 Drizzle the vinaigrette over the kale and toss well.

7 Serve with a high-quality protein.

BLT Salad Remixed

Everyone loves a good BLT—and this recipe allows you to enjoy all the great flavors of a BLT without the inflammatory ingredients that leave you feeling achy, bloated, and fatigued.

INGREDIENTS

6-8 strips humanely raised bacon, cooked and diced

6 cups mixed greens or red leaf lettuce, coarsely chopped

1 cup cherry or grape tomatoes, halved

½ cup blue cheese crumbles

1 avocado, sliced

⅓ small red onion, thinly sliced

⅓ English hothouse cucumber, diced

¼ teaspoon garlic powder

Salt and pepper, to taste

⅓ cup Ranch Dressing (see recipe on page 89)

INSTRUCTIONS

1 Preheat the oven to 375°F.

2 Line the bacon on a baking sheet pan and cook in the oven for about 18 to 20 minutes.

3 While the bacon is cooking, prep the salad greens, tomatoes, blue cheese, avocado, onion, and cucumber. Combine the salad ingredients in a large bowl.

4 Add the garlic powder and desired salt and pepper to the salad. Remember not to add too much salt since the bacon has enough flavor.

5 Once the bacon has finished cooking, let it cool on a separate plate lined with a paper towel.

6 Coarsely chop the cooled bacon and add it to the salad.

7 Toss the salad with desired dressing or homemade Ranch Dressing.

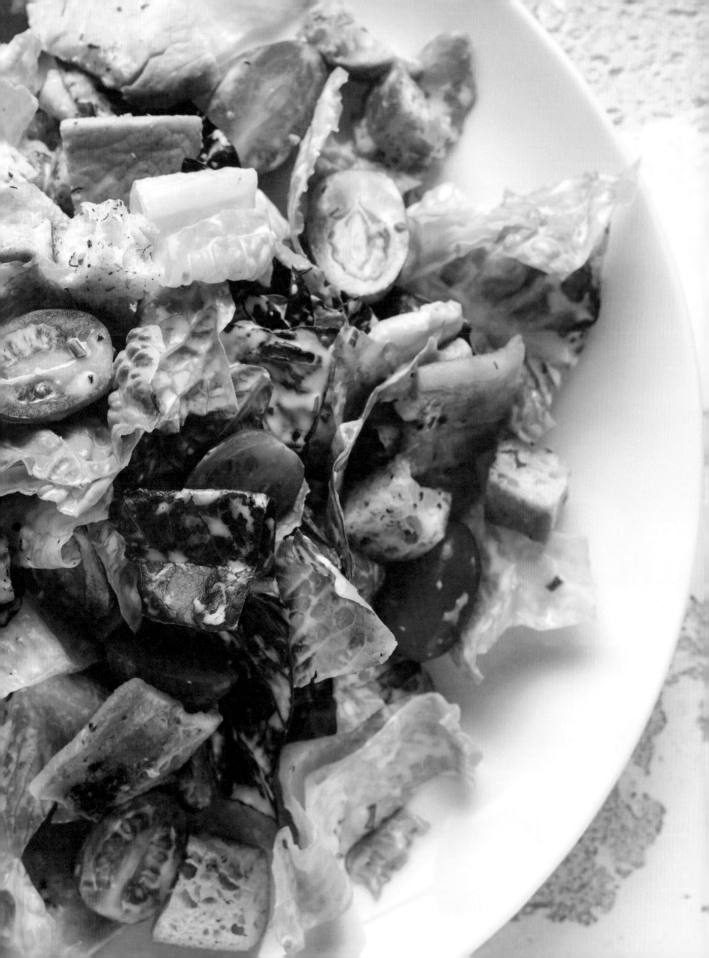

Krissy's Famous Taco Salad

This is a fun and tasty salad that's easy to make for a quick meal. It's filled with complex carbs and high-quality protein and fat to keep you fueled and full. To keep this recipe anti-inflammatory, pay attention to the quality of your ingredients. If you're sensitive to dairy, replace the cheese with 1½ tablespoons of nutritional yeast.

INGREDIENTS

1 lb. pasture-raised ground beef

2 tablespoons Taco Seasoning (see recipe on page 97)

6 cups mixed greens or red leaf lettuce, coarsely chopped

1 cup vine tomatoes, diced

⅓ red onion, diced

1 red bell pepper, diced

⅓ cup crushed tortilla chips (I like to use Siete chips)

⅓ cup shredded Cheddar cheese from pasture-raised cows (optional, I like to use Horizon)

1 medium avocado, cubed

⅓ cup Homemade Salsa (see recipe on page 102)

⅓ cup Ranch Dressing (see recipe on page 89)

INSTRUCTIONS

1 Heat oil in a skillet over medium-high heat. Add ground beef and break it apart with a spatula.

2 Sprinkle meat with Taco Seasoning. Toss to combine. Continue cooking the beef, occasionally breaking large chunks with a spatula. Cook for about 10 to 13 minutes, until the beef is browned and the moisture has evaporated.

3 While the beef is cooking, combine the greens, tomatoes, onion, red bell pepper, tortilla chips, cheese, and avocado.

4 Combine the Homemade Salsa and Ranch Dressing together and pour over salad. Toss to combine.

5 Once the beef has finished cooking, add it to the salad, toss again, and serve.

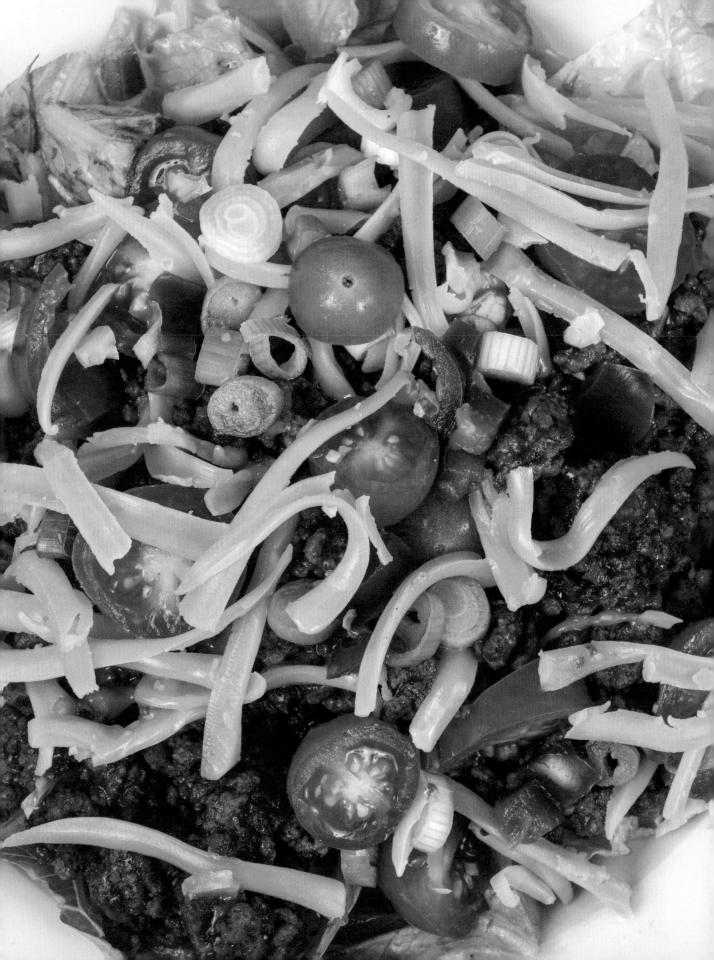

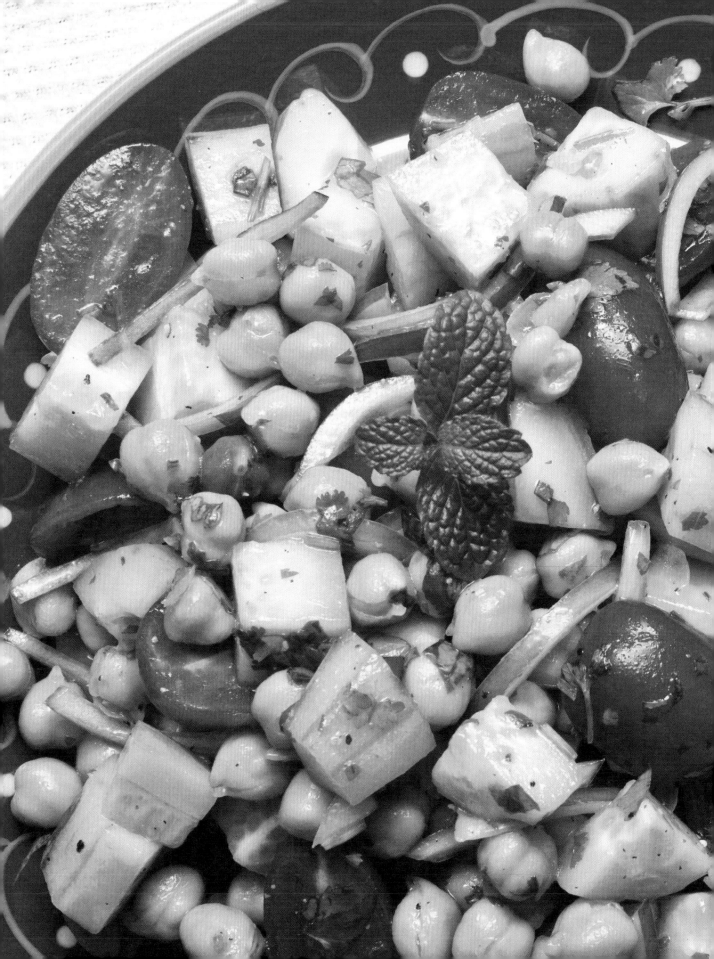

Refreshing Summer Salad

Contrary to the name, this salad is so good you can have it any time of year! Garbanzo beans are packed with fiber, selenium, magnesium, calcium, potassium, B vitamins, and iron. These nutrients reduce and prevent inflammation and support heart health while the fat, protein, and fiber content will keep you fueled and energized to tackle the rest of your day.

INGREDIENTS

2 medium English cucumbers, chopped

1 medium tomato, chopped

½ cup diced red onion

1 cup garbanzo beans, drained and rinsed

⅓ cup chopped cilantro

2 tablespoons red wine vinegar

2 tablespoons lemon juice

3 tablespoons extra-virgin olive oil

¼ teaspoon garlic powder

¼ teaspoon salt

¼ teaspoon black pepper

1 medium avocado, chopped

INSTRUCTIONS

1 Add all ingredients to a bowl and toss until well combined.

Crunchy Honey-Mustard Salad

This is one cruciferous superfood salad! This delicious salad is full of selenium, vitamin C, tocopherols, folate, calcium, and zinc. These nutrients support your immune system, minimize inflammation, and help prevent chronic diseases.

INGREDIENTS

4 cups broccoli florets, chopped to about the size of a quarter

2 cups radishes, sliced thin

1 cup slivered almonds or pecans, lightly toasted

⅓ cup red onion, thinly sliced

½ cup dried cranberries

Dressing

⅔ cup extra-virgin olive oil

¼ cup apple cider vinegar

2 tablespoons Dijon mustard

2 tablespoons raw honey

¼ teaspoon fine sea salt

INSTRUCTIONS

1 In a large mixing bowl, combine the broccoli florets, radishes, almonds, red onion, and dried cranberries.

2 In a separate bowl, combine the dressing ingredients and whisk until well combined.

3 Pour the dressing over the salad ingredients and toss.

4 For best results, let the salad sit for about 40 minutes to 1 hour before serving.

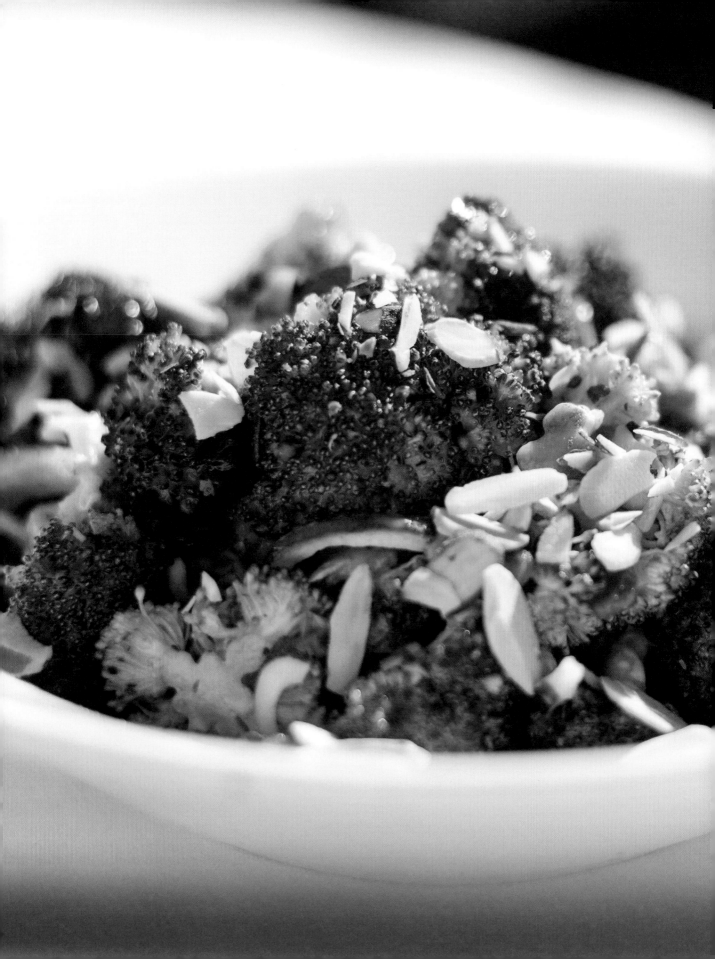

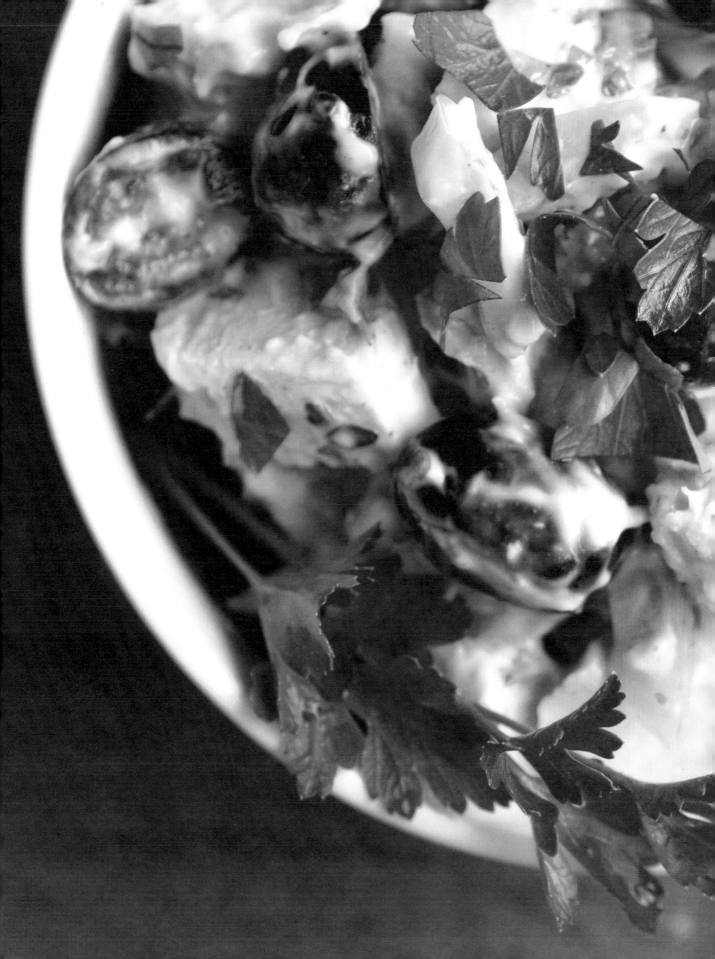

Dairy-Free Chicken Salad

This delicious chicken salad is dairy-free to help avoid inflammation associated with dairy consumption. You can eat it alone, in a lettuce wrap, or add to a salad for protein.

INGREDIENTS

2 cups rotisserie or leftover chicken, shredded

¼ cup roasted almonds, chopped

1½ cups seedless red grapes, halved

2 medium stalks celery, diced

½ cup scallions, chopped

⅓ green bell pepper, diced

2 tablespoons fresh dill, chopped

1 tablespoon fresh parsley, chopped

¼ cup tahini

3 tablespoons hot water

1 tablespoon lemon juice

1 tablespoon apple cider vinegar

Salt and pepper, to taste

¼ teaspoon garlic powder, plus more to taste

INSTRUCTIONS

1 In a large mixing bowl, combine the chicken, almonds, grapes, celery, scallions, bell pepper, dill, and fresh parsley.

2 In a small mixing bowl, whisk the tahini, hot water, lemon juice, apple cider vinegar, salt, pepper, and garlic powder until well combined and smooth.

3 Add the dressing to the salad bowl and toss well to combine. Adjust the seasoning as needed.

Roasted Brussels Sprouts

This dish is simple, delicious, and rich in nutrients that help rid your body of pro-inflammatory toxins.

INGREDIENTS

1 lb. Brussels sprouts, ends trimmed, washed, and halved

2 tablespoons extra-virgin olive oil

½ teaspoon sea salt

½ teaspoon black pepper

1 tablespoon onion powder

1 tablespoon grass-fed butter

1 small onion, sliced thin

⅓ cup roasted pistachios, roughly chopped

INSTRUCTIONS

1 Preheat oven to 400°F.

2 Place the Brussels sprouts on a large sheet pan. Add the olive oil, salt, pepper, and onion powder. Toss well with tongs or clean hands.

3 Roast in the pan in the oven for about 15 to 20 minutes or until the Brussels sprouts are tender and golden brown. Toss once or twice as they're roasting.

4 While the Brussels sprouts are roasting, heat butter in a skillet. Once the butter is melted, add the sliced onions and sauté for about 8 to 10 minutes or until onions become translucent and aromatic.

5 Add the roasted pistachios to the Brussels sprouts when there are about 2 minutes of roasting time remaining.

6 Once the Brussels sprouts and pistachios are done, remove them from the oven and add them to the pan with the onions.

7 Sauté everything together for about 2 minutes, then serve.

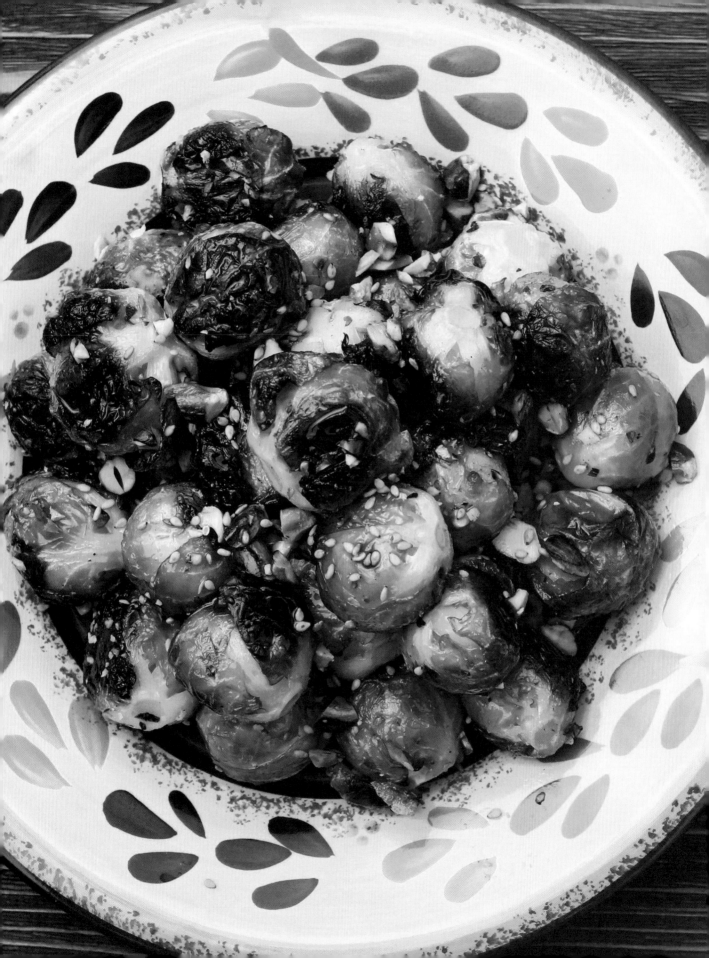

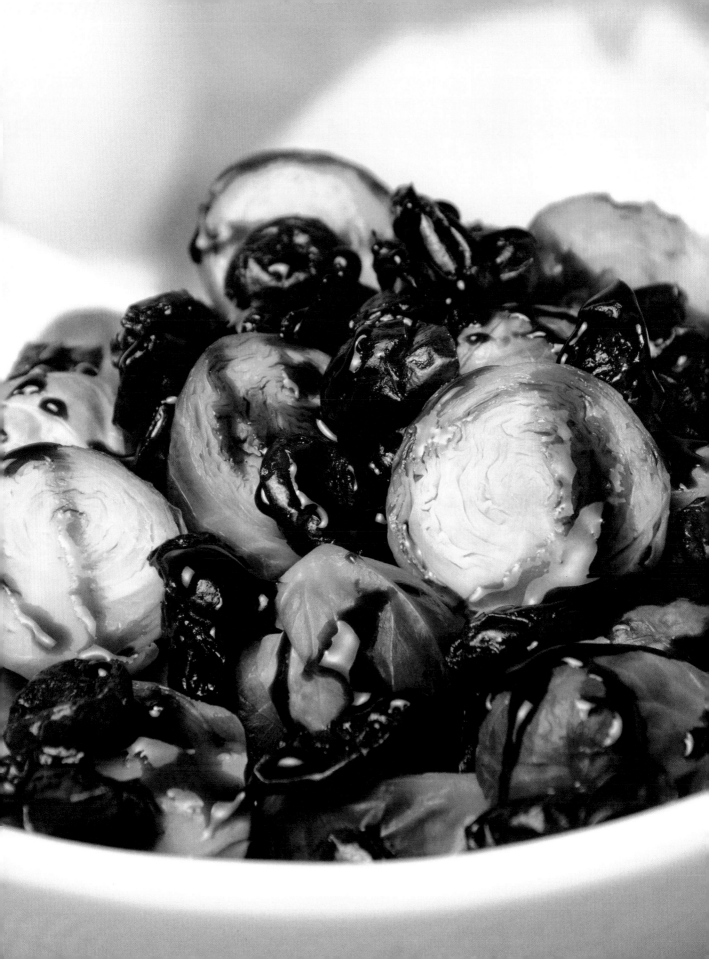

Balsamic Glazed Brussels Sprouts

This sweet and savory side dish pairs nicely with grilled steak, chicken, or fish. Brussels sprouts are a great source of vitamin C and K and are guaranteed to appeal to even the pickiest eater.

INGREDIENTS

4 cups Brussels sprouts, split in half lengthwise

2 tablespoons olive oil

½ teaspoon salt

¼ teaspoon black pepper

¾ cup balsamic vinegar

2 tablespoons raw honey or maple syrup

¼ cup dried cranberries

¼ cup feta cheese (omit if sensitive to dairy)

INSTRUCTIONS

1   Preheat the oven to 400°F.

2   Place the Brussels sprouts on a baking sheet. Toss with olive oil, salt, and pepper.

3   Place the baking sheet in the oven for 20 to 25 minutes or until the Brussels sprouts are golden brown.

4   While the Brussels sprouts are cooking, pour balsamic vinegar and honey into a saucepan. Bring the sauce to a boil and reduce it to a simmer for about 10 to 13 minutes or until the vinegar reduces and begins to thicken.

5   Take the baking sheet out of the oven and pour the glaze over the Brussels sprouts.

6   Toss the Brussels sprouts with cranberries and feta cheese, then serve.

Honey Mustard Brussels Sprouts

Another great Brussels sprouts recipe! Not only do these Brussels sprouts taste great but they also have a phytochemical called glucosinolate that helps reduce inflammation and eliminate toxins from your body.

INGREDIENTS

3 cups Brussels sprouts, split in half lengthwise

1 tablespoon olive oil

Salt and pepper, to taste

2 tablespoons ghee, melted

1½ tablespoons Dijon mustard

1 tablespoon raw honey

INSTRUCTIONS

1   Preheat the oven to 400°F.

2   Place the Brussels sprouts on a baking sheet. Toss with olive oil, salt, and pepper. Place the sheet into the oven for about 12 minutes.

3   While Brussels sprouts are cooking, whisk the ghee, mustard, and honey.

4   After the sprouts have been cooking for 12 minutes, remove the baking sheet from the oven and mix the sprouts into the honey-mustard mixture. Toss well with tongs and put the sheet back in the oven.

5   Cook the Brussels sprouts for another 8 to 10 minutes, then serve.

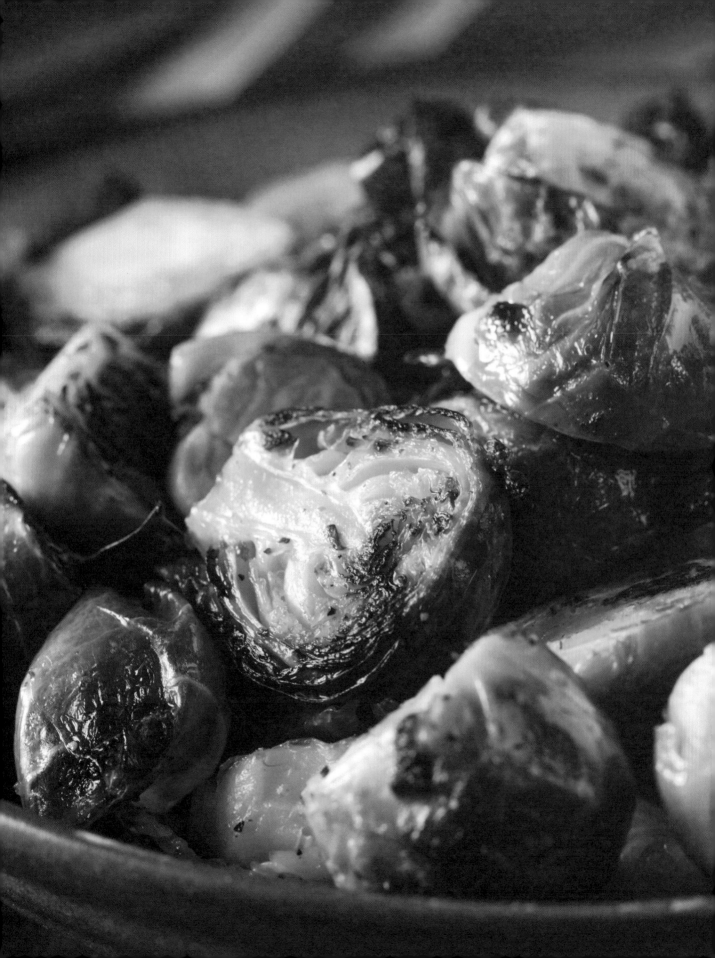

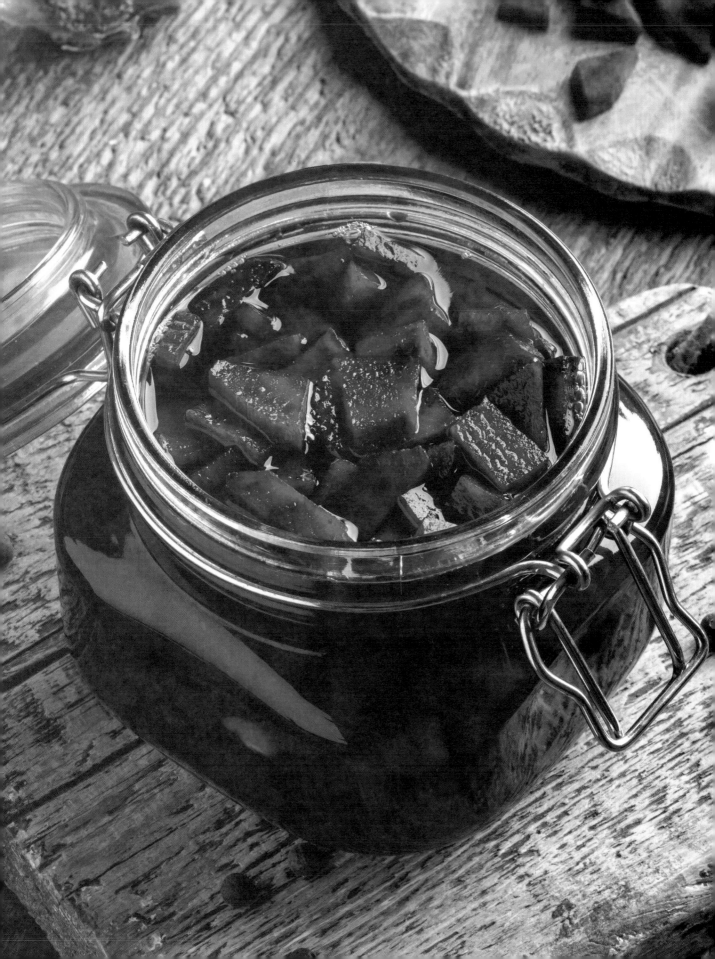

Pickled Beets

Pickled foods are incredibly anti-inflammatory and delicious. They contain bacteria that not only support our gut health but also reduce any cravings for inflammatory foods. Beets are packed with fiber, B vitamins, and potassium that help minimize inflammation within our bodies.

INGREDIENTS

5 beets

¼ cup apple cider vinegar

1 tablespoon coconut sugar

1 tablespoon extra-virgin olive oil

½ teaspoon dry mustard

¼ teaspoon salt

¼ teaspoon black pepper

INSTRUCTIONS

1 Place the beets in a medium saucepan and cover with water. Bring to a boil and maintain a simmer for 30 to 40 minutes, or until the beets become tender and you are easily able to pierce them with a fork.

2 After the beets are done cooking, place them in a strainer and run cold water over them. Use your fingers to peel the skin off of the beets and slice them to your desired thickness.

3 Combine the apple cider vinegar, coconut sugar, olive oil, dry mustard, salt, and pepper in a small bowl and whisk. Adjust seasonings needed.

4 Combine beets and vinaigrette in a mason jar and leave at room temperature for about an hour.

5 Store in the fridge until ready to eat.

Spanish Cauliflower Rice

If you're opting for a lower carb option than rice, this is a great alternative.
It's full of flavor and micronutrients to keep your body functioning at its best.

INGREDIENTS

1 large head cauliflower

2 tablespoons avocado oil

½ cup diced yellow onion

4 garlic cloves, minced

1 teaspoon cumin

1 teaspoon oregano

1 teaspoon garlic powder

½ teaspoon salt

1 tablespoon tomato paste

¼ cup chicken broth

¼ cup cilantro, chopped

Juice of ½ lime

½ teaspoon lime zest

INSTRUCTIONS

1 Cut the cauliflower head into quarters. Remove the large stem and place the cauliflower into the food processor. You may need to place a quarter of the cauliflower into the processor at a time for the cauliflower to reach a rice consistency.

2 Heat the avocado oil in a large skillet. Add the onions and garlic and sauté for about 3 minutes or until the onion and garlic become fragrant.

3 Add the cauliflower rice along with cumin, oregano, garlic powder, and salt. Sauté for about 4 to 6 minutes.

4 Toss in the tomato paste and chicken broth. Sauté until the tomato paste is well integrated into the rice.

5 Stir in the cilantro, lime juice, and lime zest. Stir for about 1 to 2 more minutes.

6 Remove the skillet from the heat and serve immediately.

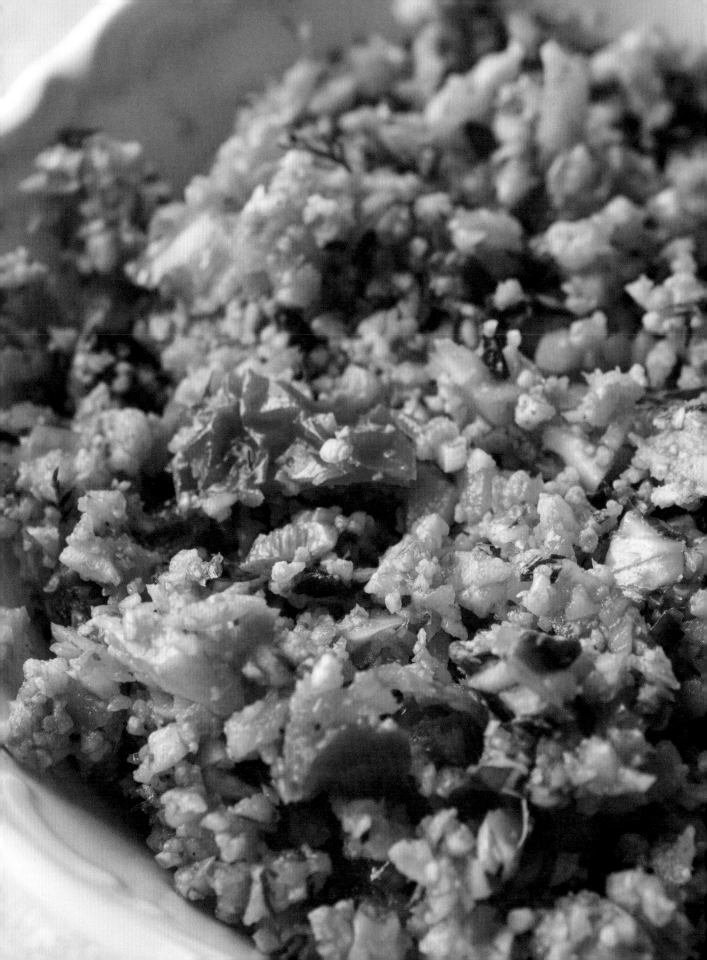

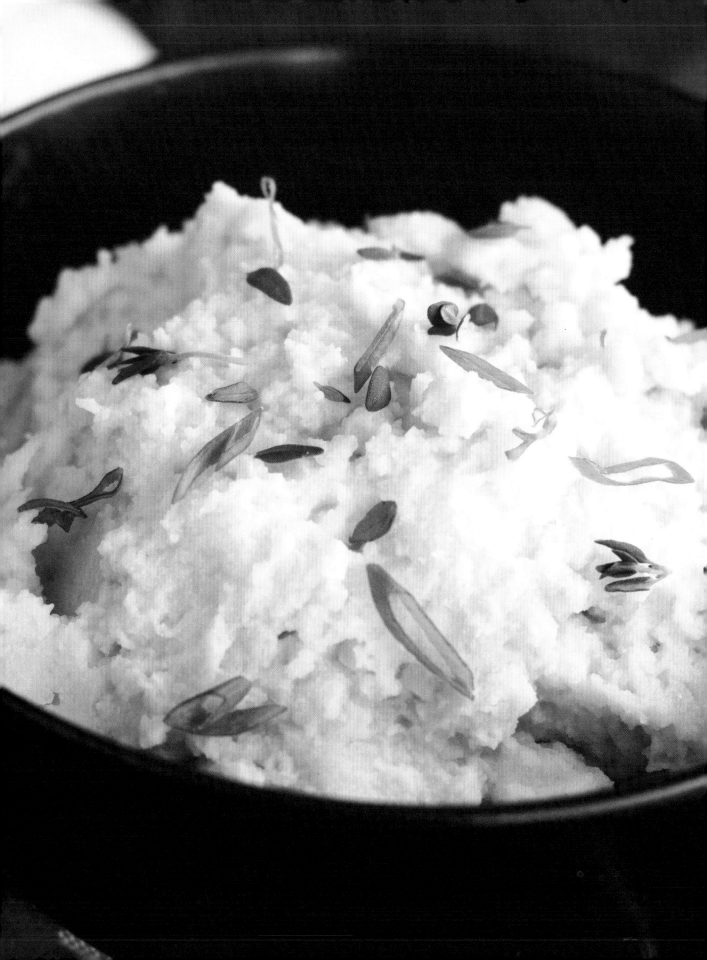

Cauliflower Mash

When trying to incorporate anti-inflammatory foods into your diet, you need to be a bit creative. This recipe uses cauliflower in place of the more traditional mashed potato. Cauliflower gives you more bang for your buck in terms of nutrients and you won't be able to tell the difference from your traditional mash!

INGREDIENTS

1 medium head cauliflower, chopped, large stems removed

1 tablespoon olive oil

½ cup coconut cream

½ teaspoon sea salt

¼ teaspoon garlic powder

1 teaspoon chives

3 tablespoons grass-fed butter

INSTRUCTIONS

1 Preheat the oven to 425°F.

2 Place the cauliflower florets on a baking sheet and coat with olive oil.

3 Roast the cauliflower for 15 minutes, or until cauliflower is fork-tender.

4 Remove the baking sheet from the oven. Add the roasted cauliflower and the remaining ingredients into a food processor and process until smooth.

Herb Roasted Sweet Potatoes

The fresh herbs of these delicious sweet potatoes not only carry numerous vitamins and minerals, they also contain different polyphenols that support health and protect against chronic diseases.

INGREDIENTS

2 medium sweet potatoes, peeled and cubed

2 sprigs fresh rosemary, chopped

1 sprig fresh thyme, chopped

½ teaspoon Italian seasoning

2 tablespoons olive oil

1 tablespoon garlic powder

1 tablespoon salt

1 tablespoon black pepper

Cooking spray

INSTRUCTIONS

1 Preheat oven to 425°F.

2 In a medium-sized mixing bowl, combine the ingredients and toss well to coat.

3 Lightly spray a baking sheet with cooking spray and place the potatoes on the tray.

4 Place the pan in the oven and roast for about 30 minutes or until the potatoes are golden brown and fork-tender.

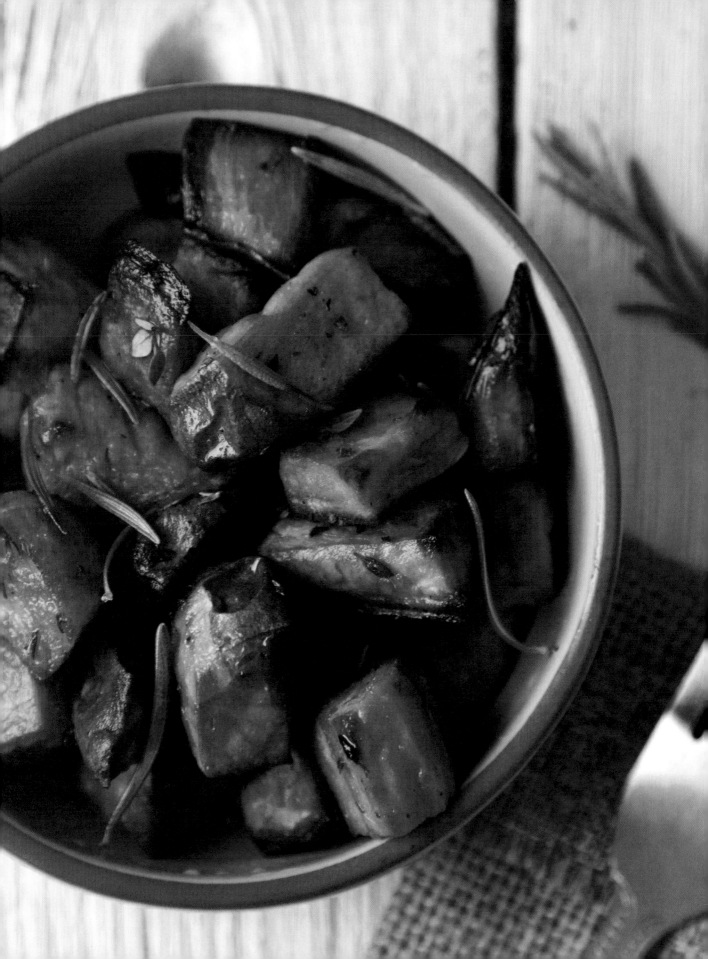

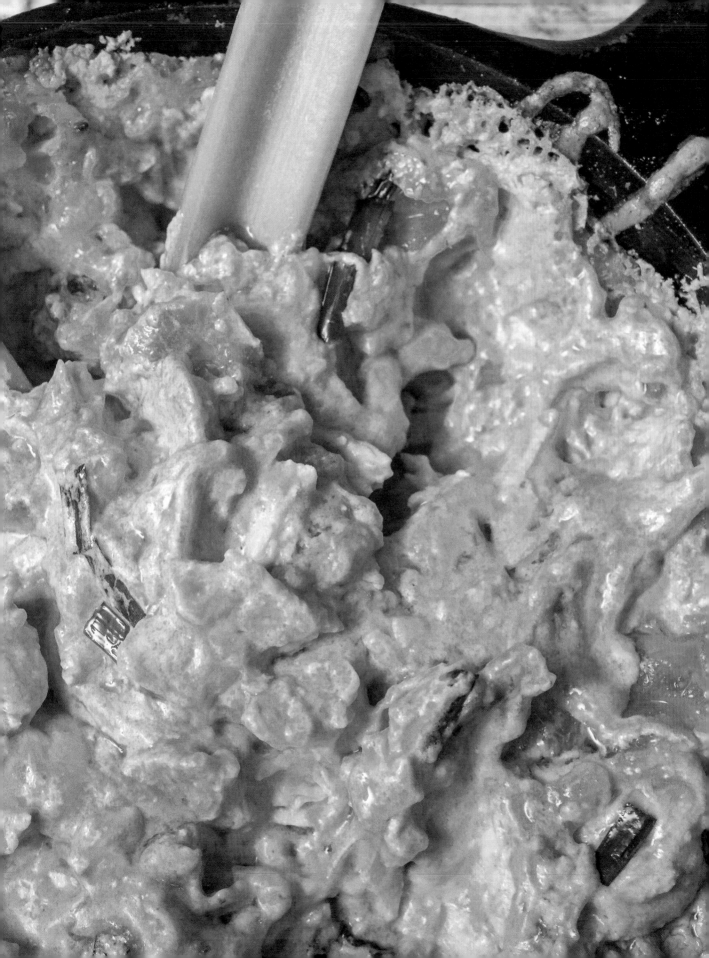

Chicken Buffalo Dip

This recipe is the perfect game-day addition. Being successful in your health goals means finding food you genuinely love and can incorporate into your lifestyle. This nutrient-dense dip is one that can be enjoyed by the whole family.

INGREDIENTS

1 medium sweet potato, baked

½ cup full-fat coconut milk

¼ cup Frank's Red Hot Sauce

3 tablespoons nutritional yeast

1 tablespoon extra-virgin olive oil

1 teaspoon sea salt

1 teaspoon garlic powder

1 teaspoon onion powder

1 cup rotisserie chicken, shredded

⅓ cup blue cheese (optional)

INSTRUCTIONS

1 In a blender or food processor, add the flesh of the baked sweet potato. You can also use leftover sweet potato mash here.

2 Add the coconut milk, hot sauce, nutritional yeast, olive oil, salt, garlic powder, and onion powder. Blend until smooth.

3 In a large serving dish, add the dip from the blender along with the shredded chicken. Mix to combine.

4 Top with the blue cheese if you're not sensitive to dairy. If desired, place the dish in the oven at 375°F for 10 minutes.

Honey-Lemon Dressing

This is a great dressing to use on any salad. What keeps this recipe anti-inflammatory is the use of raw honey. Raw honey has all of the vitamins and phytonutrients you need to support your immune system's efforts in reducing inflammation. These nutrients are usually lost or damaged with conventionally bought honey.

INGREDIENTS

⅓ cup fresh lemon juice

2 teaspoons lemon zest

3 tablespoons basil, minced

2 tablespoons raw honey

2 tablespoons olive oil

Salt and pepper, to taste

INSTRUCTIONS

1 Whisk all of the ingredients together in an airtight container until well combined.

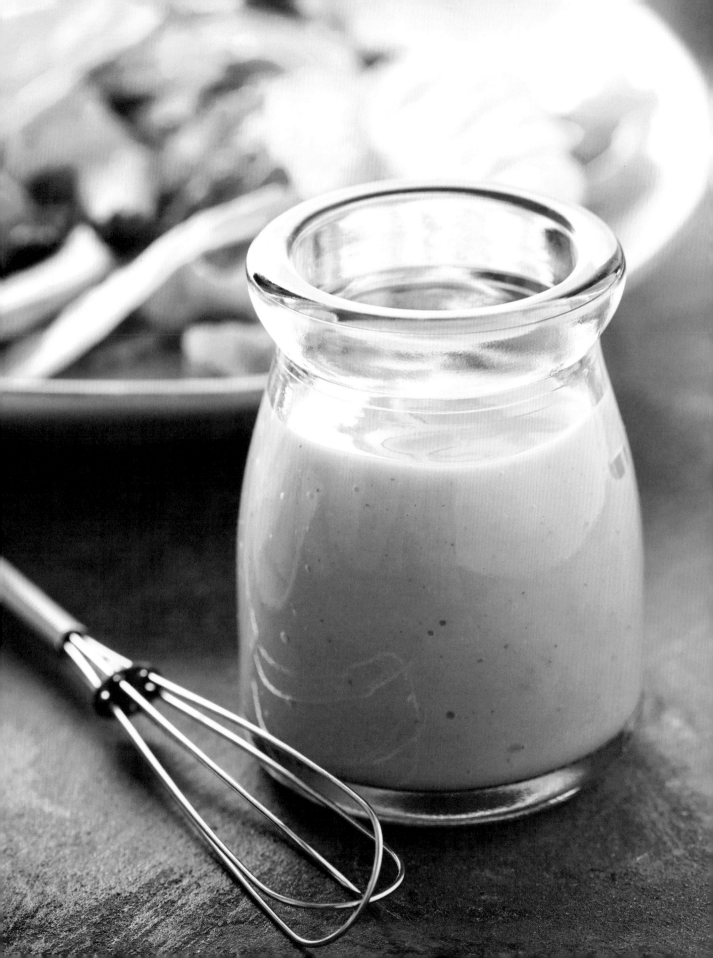

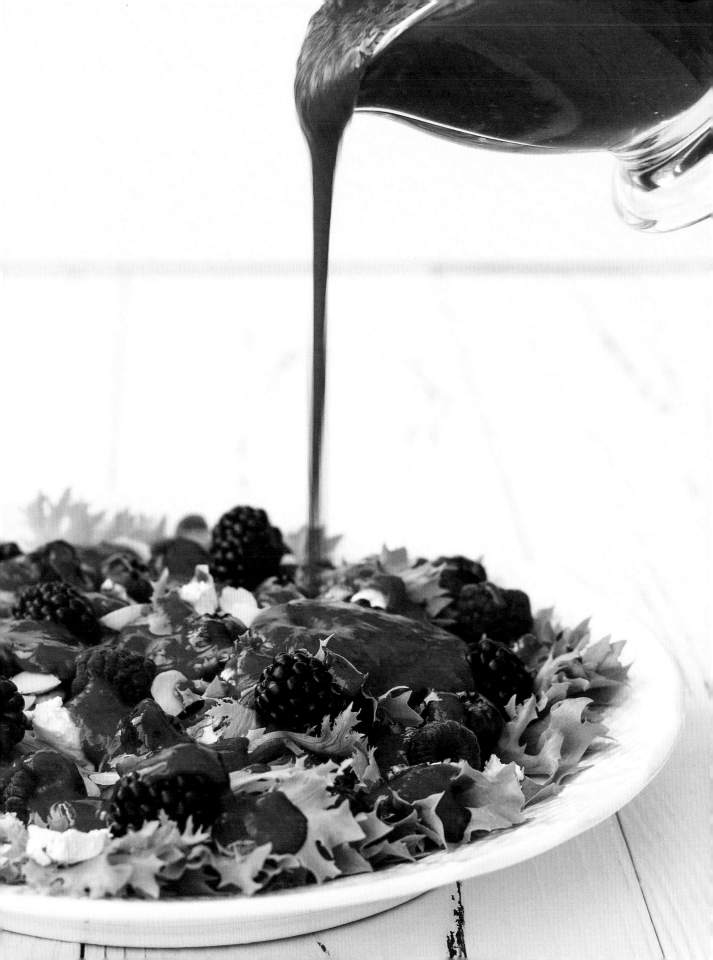

Cranberry Honey Dressing

Oddly enough, some people think salads are exclusively for warmer weather. This recipe proves them wrong. The warm spices in this dressing will perfectly complement your favorite nutrient-packed salads any time of the year.

INGREDIENTS

¼ cup fresh cranberries

2 tablespoons raw honey

3 tablespoons apple cider vinegar

½ teaspoon ground mustard

1½ teaspoons shallots

¼ cup avocado oil

Pinch of allspice

Salt and pepper, to taste

INSTRUCTIONS

1   Place all of the ingredients in a food processor or blender and blend until smooth.

Turmeric Tahini Dressing

Packed with warm spices and ingredients rich in antioxidants and phytonutrients, this dressing is guaranteed to help support your immune system and natural ability to detox.

INGREDIENTS

¼ cup tahini

¼ cup lemon juice

2 tablespoons water

1 tablespoon olive oil

1 tablespoon nutritional yeast

½ tablespoon maple syrup
or raw honey

¼ teaspoon sea salt

¼ teaspoon black pepper

¼ teaspoon ground turmeric

¼ teaspoon garlic powder

1 tablespoon freshly grated
ginger

INSTRUCTIONS

1　Place all ingredients in a small bowl. Whisk until well combined and smooth.

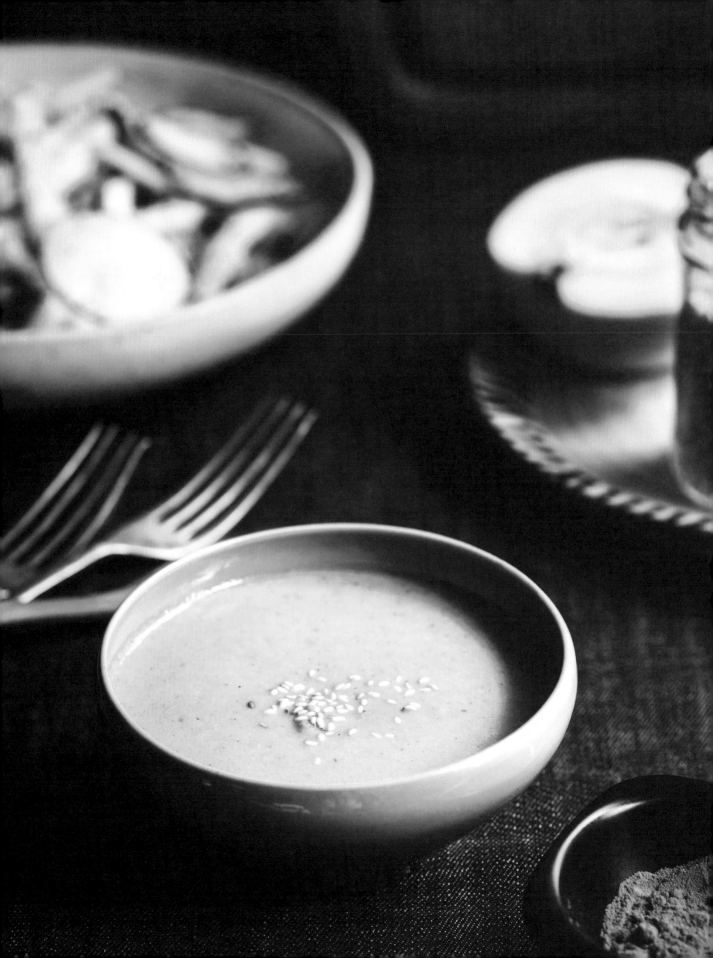

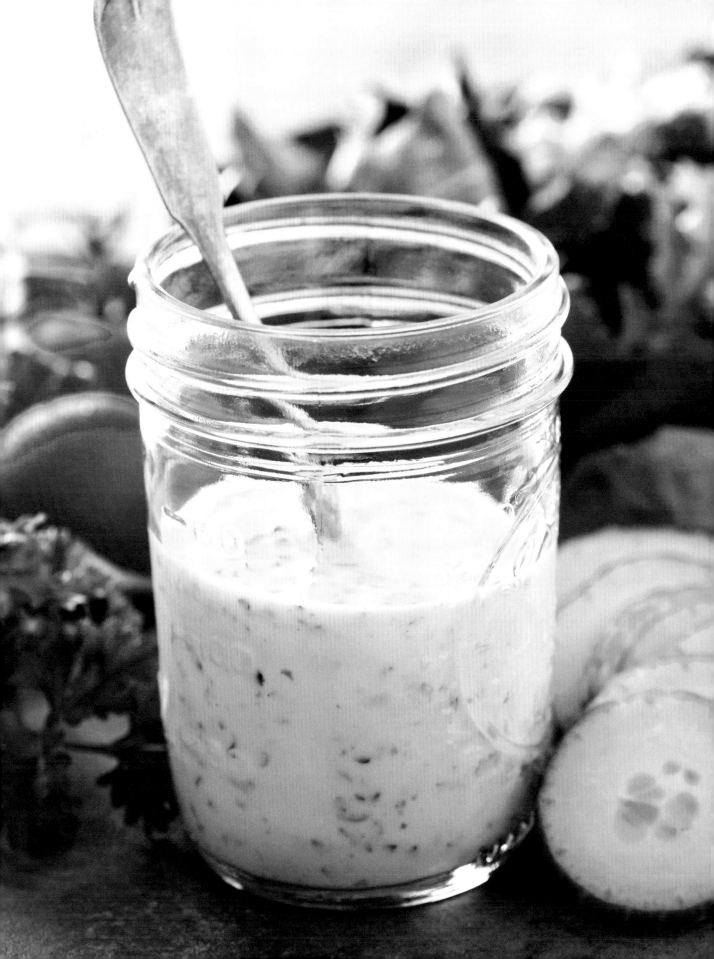

Ranch Dressing

This is a great replacement for your typical ranch dressing because it omits the inflammatory hydrogenated oils, preservatives, and sugars without compromising great flavor.

INGREDIENTS

⅓ cup Paleo mayonnaise (I like to use Primal Kitchen Mayo)

¼ cup canned full-fat coconut milk

1 tablespoon dried parsley

1 tablespoon dried chives

1 teaspoon dried dill

1 teaspoon garlic powder

1 teaspoon onion powder

½ teaspoon apple cider vinegar

½ teaspoon sea salt

¼ teaspoon black pepper

INSTRUCTIONS

1 Place all ingredients in a blender and blend on the lowest setting until well combined. You may also place all of the ingredients in a bowl and whisk until well combined.

2 Place in refrigerator for at least 30 minutes before serving.

Greek Salad Dressing

Everyone loves a good Greek salad. Unfortunately, store-bought dressings have lots of inflammatory sugars and partially hydrogenated oils. With this delicious homemade option, you'll find plenty of anti-inflammatory compounds and nutrients from garlic, oregano, and olive oil that quiet inflammatory immune responses, minimize oxidative stress, and support heart health.

INGREDIENTS

4 garlic cloves, minced

2 teaspoons dried oregano

1 teaspoon Dijon mustard

½ cup red wine vinegar

2 teaspoons sea salt

1 teaspoon black pepper

1 cup extra-virgin olive oil

INSTRUCTIONS

1 Place all of the ingredients in a small bowl and whisk until well combined.

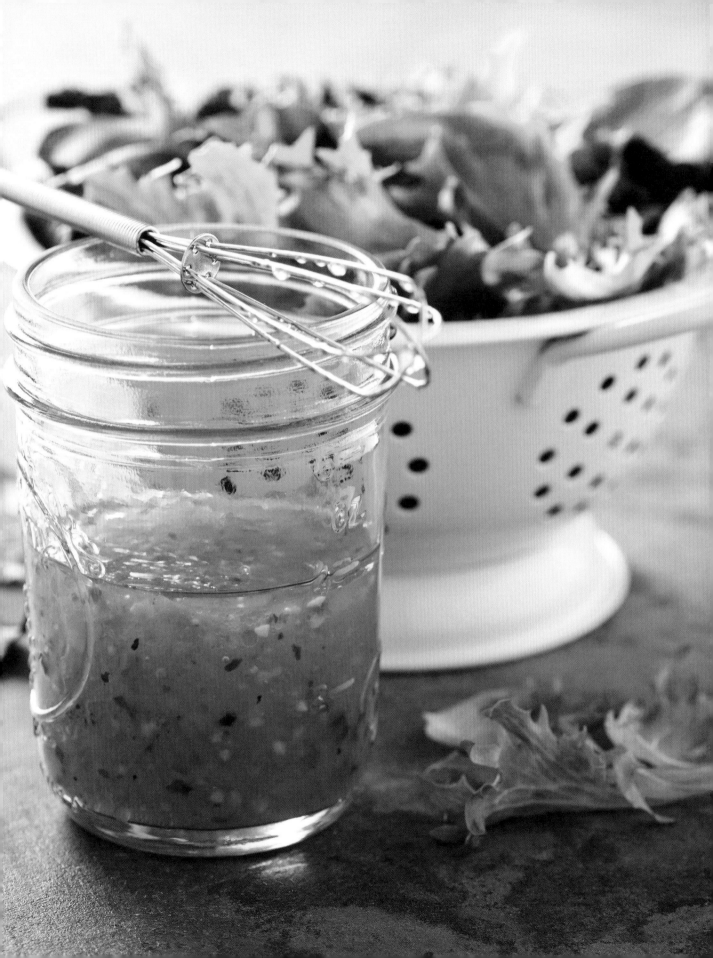

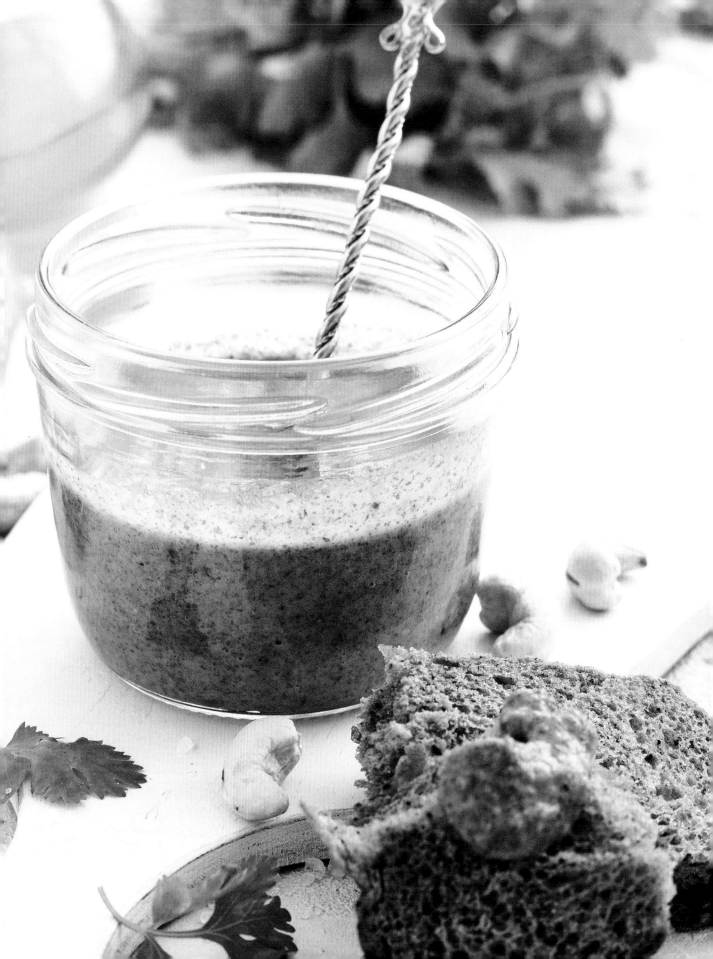

Cilantro-Lime Vinaigrette

This dressing goes perfectly with any Latin-inspired salad. Lime is rich in the antioxidant vitamin C, which helps your body fight off any potential inflammatory triggers. Lime juice also raises your stomach's pH levels, which will help you absorb essential minerals, digest your food properly, and avoid possible inflammatory triggers during the digestion process.

INGREDIENTS

⅓ cup extra-virgin olive oil or avocado oil

3 tablespoons freshly-squeezed lime juice

1 tablespoon apple cider vinegar

2 teaspoons raw honey

1 teaspoon garlic salt

¼ cup cilantro, chopped

1 teaspoon dried oregano

Sea salt and black pepper, to taste

INSTRUCTIONS

1 For best results, add all of the ingredients into a food processor and process until smooth. You may also mince the cilantro and combine all of the ingredients in a small bowl and whisk until well combined.

Anti-Inflammatory Caesar Salad Dressing

Everyone loves Caesar salad. However, store-bought dressings contain damaged oils and added sugars which trigger inflammation within our bodies. This recipe lets you enjoy your favorite salad without compromising your health.

INGREDIENTS

1 cup macadamia nuts or soaked cashews (soak cashews in water for 4 hours)

2 small garlic cloves

2 tablespoons nutritional yeast

2 tablespoons capers

Juice of 1 lemon

1 tablespoon coconut aminos

2 tablespoons olive oil

1 tablespoon Dijon mustard

½ teaspoon garlic powder

Salt and pepper, to taste

¼ cup water

INSTRUCTIONS

1 Add all of the dressing ingredients except the water to a blender.

2 Add water into the blender little by little to reach the desired thickness. Blend the dressing until smooth.

3 Enjoy with your favorite salad greens.

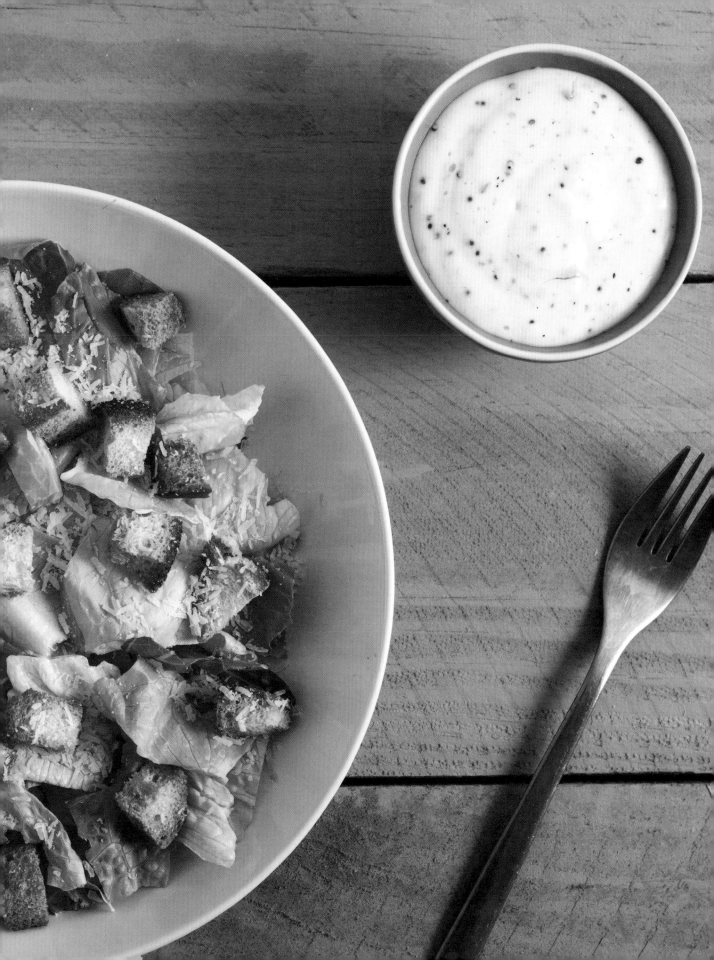

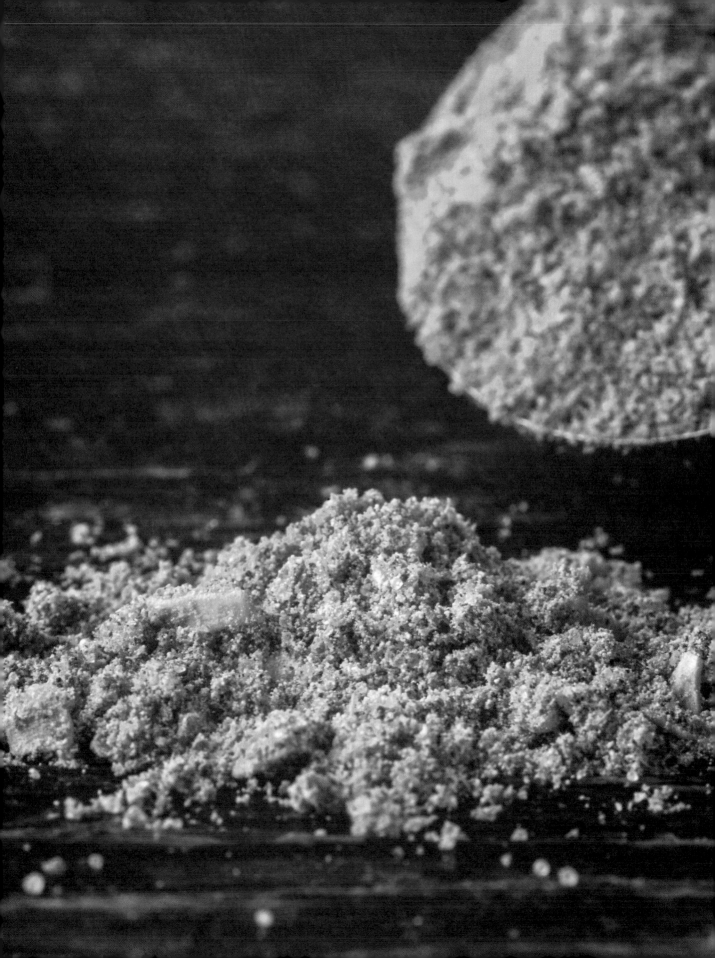

Taco Seasoning

Most store-bought seasonings have additives, preservatives, and colorings that stimulate the inflammatory pathways in our bodies. This recipe uses everyday spices to create an amazing seasoning that tastes just like the store-bought ones but leaves out the nasty additives.

INGREDIENTS

2 tablespoons chili powder

1½ tablespoons ground cumin

1 tablespoon garlic powder

½ tablespoon paprika

½ tablespoon onion powder

½ tablespoon dried oregano

1 teaspoon sea salt

½ teaspoon crushed red pepper

¼ teaspoon black pepper

INSTRUCTIONS

1 Place all of the ingredients into a small, airtight container and shake well to combine. Taste and adjust ingredients as desired. Store for later use.

Packed Pesto

This is not your average pesto. This pesto is packed with antioxidants, omega-3 fatty acids, and B vitamins which keep inflammation at bay. You can add this pesto to your favorite pasta, salad, toast, or protein of your choice.

INGREDIENTS

3 cups arugula

2 cups basil leaves

1 large ripe avocado, skin and pit removed

2 garlic cloves, peeled

⅓ cup roasted pistachios

2 tablespoons lemon juice

2 tablespoons olive oil

¼ teaspoon sea salt

¼ teaspoon black pepper

INSTRUCTIONS

1   Place all of the ingredients in a food processor or blender and blend until smooth. Add more lemon juice or salt and pepper if desired.

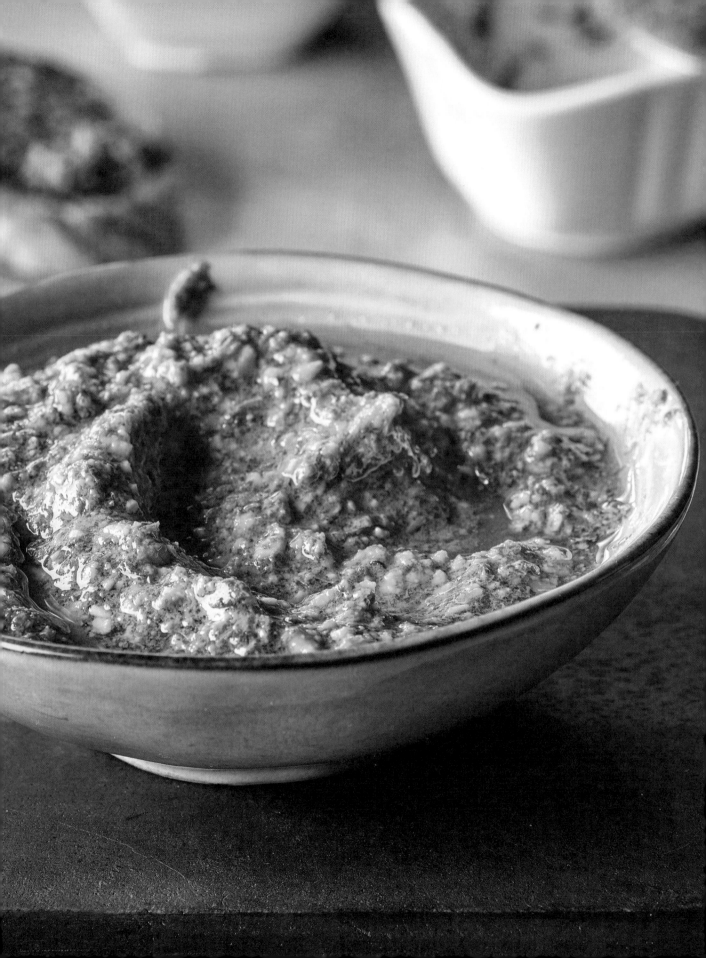

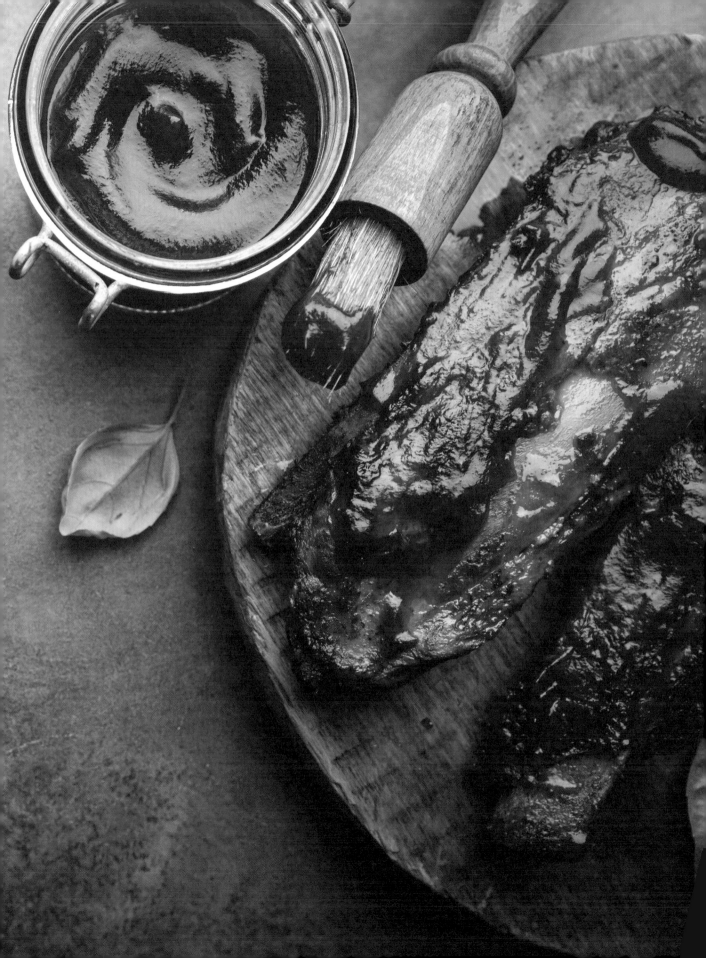

Homemade BBQ Sauce

Everyone loves BBQ sauce, but it can be full of nasty inflammatory ingredients. This BBQ sauce is made with whole foods that serve your health and avoid inflammatory responses.

INGREDIENTS

½ cup balsamic vinegar

¼-½ cup tomato sauce

1 (6 oz.) can tomato paste

6-8 pitted Medjool dates

2 tablespoons Dijon mustard

2 tablespoons coconut aminos

½ teaspoon smoked paprika

½ teaspoon garlic powder

½ teaspoon onion powder

½ teaspoon salt

½ teaspoon black pepper

INSTRUCTIONS

1 Place the ingredients into a food processor or high-speed blender and blend until smooth.

2 Transfer the blender contents into a saucepan and bring it to a simmer. Allow the mixture to simmer for about 10 to 15 minutes or until desired thickness is reached.

Homemade Salsa

Salsa isn't just for warmer weather. The heat from the spices in this nutrient-packed salsa will make you feel warm any time of year.

INGREDIENTS

4 ripe tomatoes, cored and quartered

1 red onion, peeled and quartered

3 garlic cloves, peeled

1-3 jalapeños, stemmed and seeded, to taste

⅓ cup fresh cilantro

3 tablespoons fresh lime juice

3 teaspoons ground cumin

1½ teaspoons salt

½ teaspoon garlic powder

¼ teaspoon chili powder

1 (15 oz.) can diced tomatoes

INSTRUCTIONS

1   Place all ingredients in a food processor or blender. Pulse for about a second at a time until the salsa is at the desired consistency.

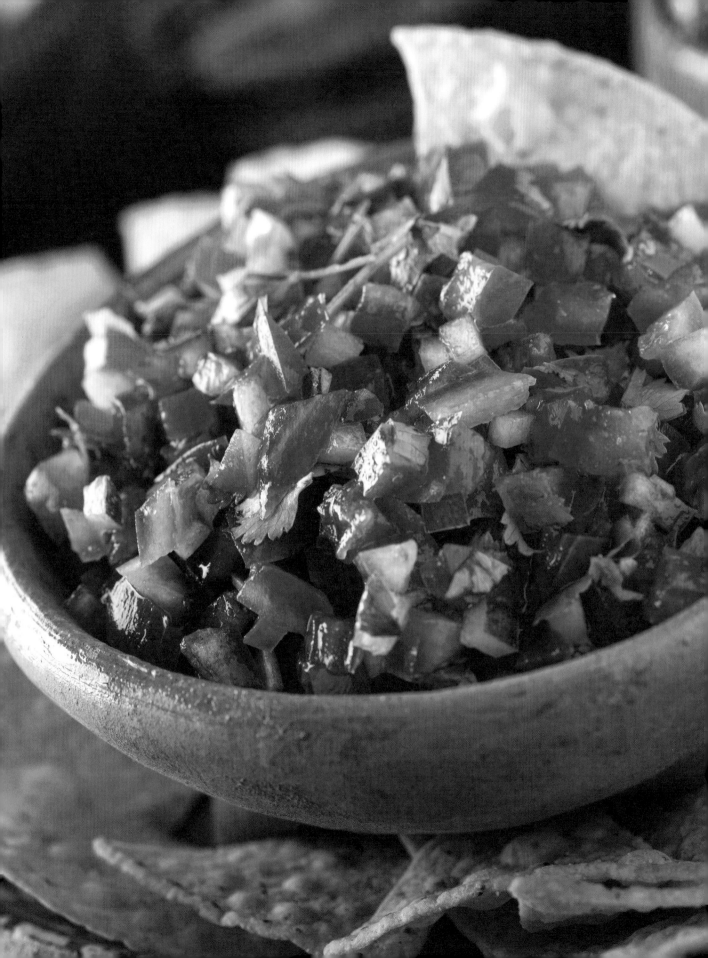

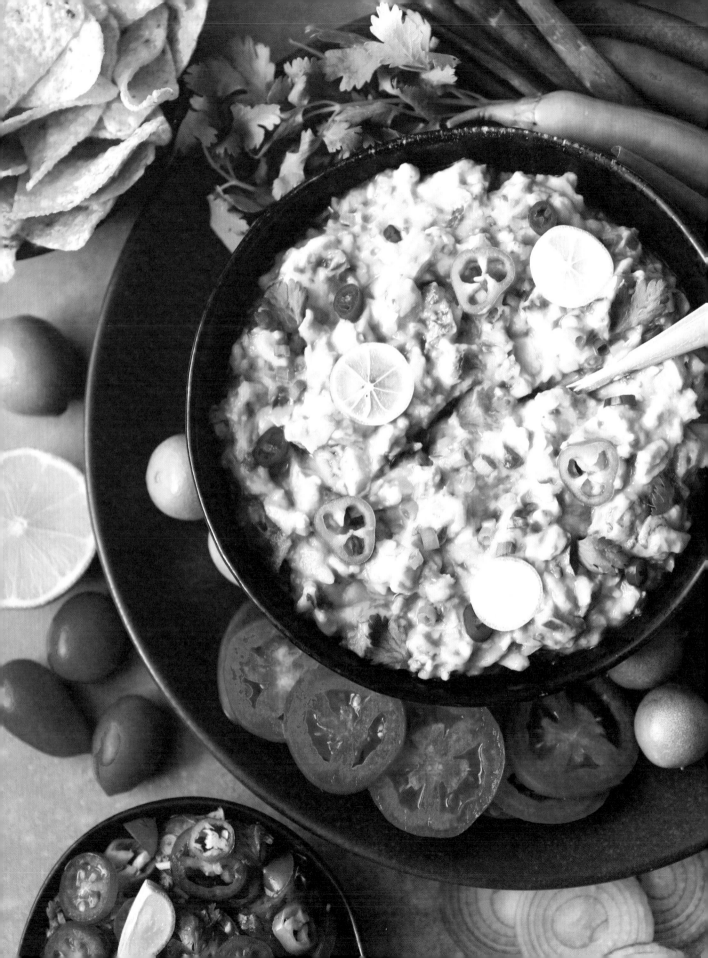

Guacamole

Guacamole is one of the best snacks anyone can have. It's rich in anti-inflammatory omega-3 fatty acids and fiber, which will help you avoid overeating at or between meals. It's also packed with several micronutrients that support your body's natural ability to eliminate waste that could otherwise cause inflammation.

INGREDIENTS

3 ripe Hass avocados, sliced open and pit removed

½ small red onion, finely diced

2 small Roma tomatoes, diced

4 tablespoons fresh cilantro, finely chopped

3-4 garlic cloves, smashed and minced

Juice of 2 limes

1 teaspoon lime zest

½ teaspoon sea salt

¼ teaspoon black pepper

¼ teaspoon garlic powder

1 jalapeño pepper, seeds removed and finely diced (optional)

INSTRUCTIONS

1   Remove the avocado from its skin and place it into a large bowl.

2   Begin mashing the avocado with a fork to your desired consistency, but leave it on the chunkier side. As you continue to mix in ingredients, the guacamole will become smoother.

3   Add the rest of the ingredients and mix until well combined.

4   Add additional salt, pepper, cilantro, or garlic powder to taste.

5   Serve with your favorite tortilla chips (opt for tortilla chips made with organic, non-GMO corn or grain-free chips).

Simple Hummus

Hummus is nutritious and versatile, and it makes a great
snack thanks to its anti-inflammatory ingredients.

INGREDIENTS

1 (15 oz.) can chickpeas, drained
and rinsed

⅓ cup tahini

2 tablespoons extra-virgin
olive oil

2 tablespoons fresh lemon juice,
plus more to taste

1 garlic clove

½ teaspoon sea salt

⅓ cup water, or as needed

1 teaspoon paprika, for garnish

INSTRUCTIONS

1 In a high-speed blender, place the chickpeas, tahini, olive
   oil, lemon juice, garlic, and salt. Process until smooth,
   adding water as needed.

2 Transfer hummus to a serving plate, top with paprika, and
   serve with vegetables.

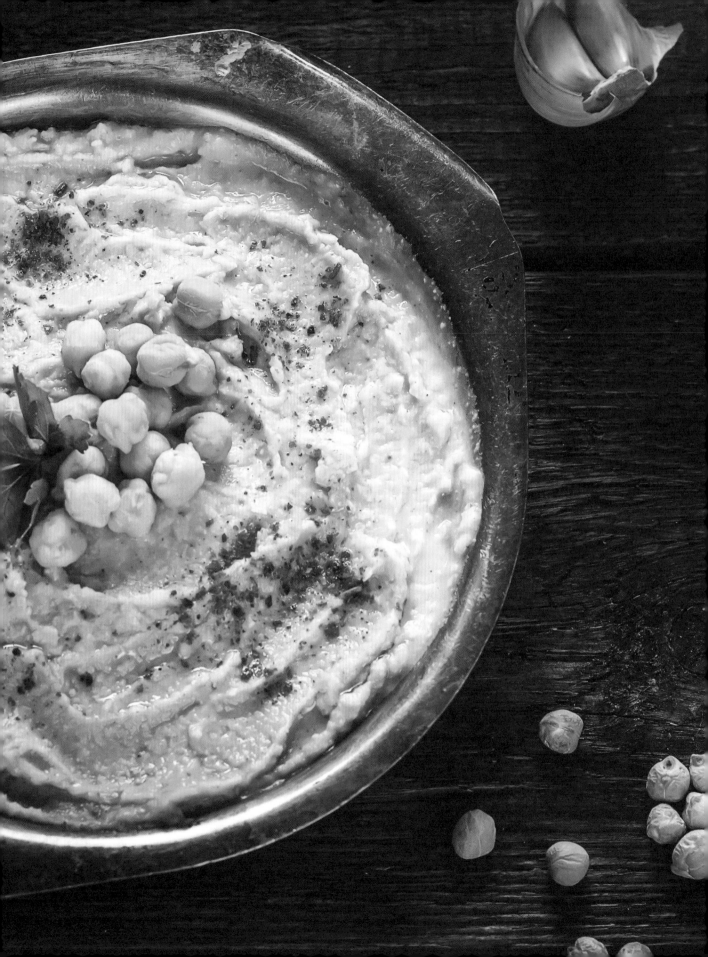

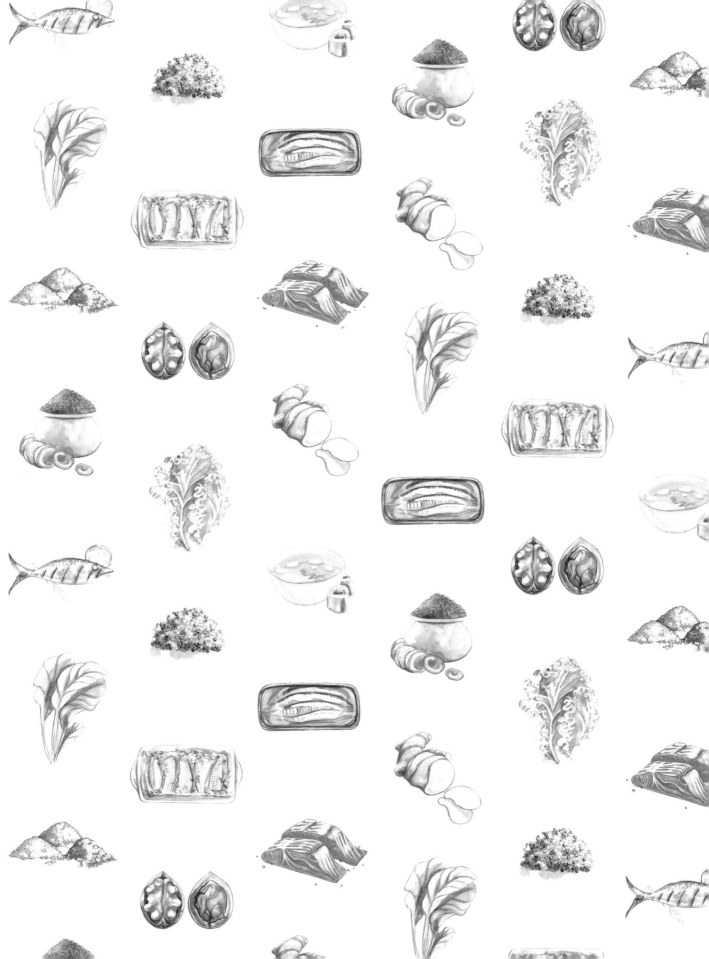

ENTREES

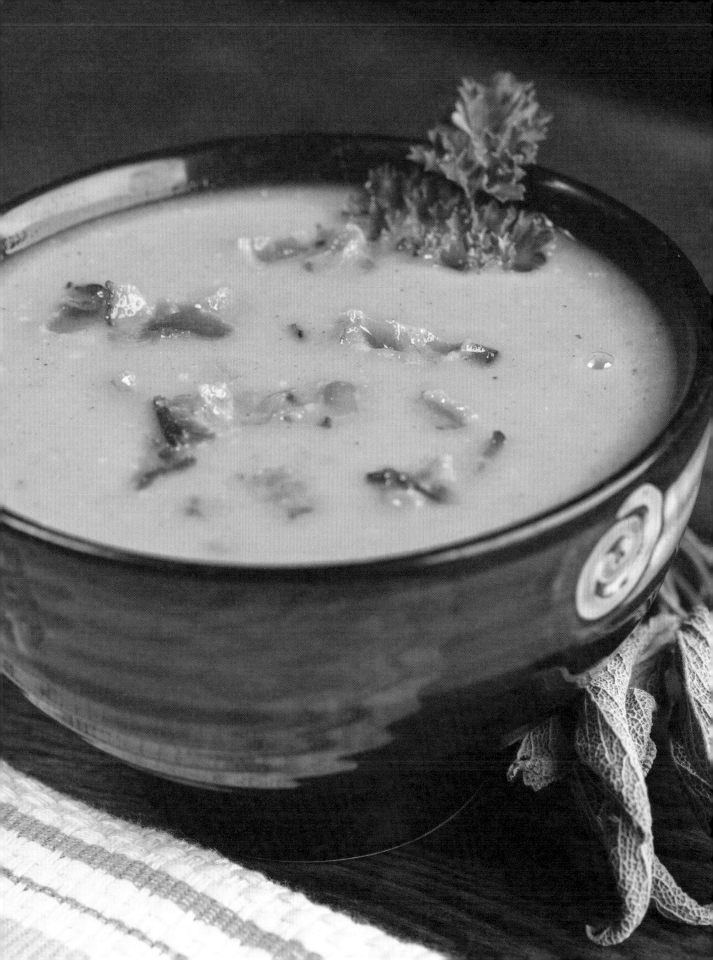

SERVINGS: 4-6 • **PREP AND COOKING TIME:** 45 MINUTES

Butternut Squash Soup

Butternut squash is packed with beta-carotene that protects your immune system from inflammation. This recipe also uses bacon and coconut, which both provide the high-quality fat you need to feel satisfied.

INGREDIENTS

5 strips humanely raised bacon, chopped

1 tablespoon olive oil

1 medium onion, chopped

3 cloves garlic, minced

1 large butternut squash, cubed

1 large apple, peeled and chopped

1½ teaspoons Italian seasoning

½ teaspoon cinnamon

½ teaspoon ginger

½ teaspoon chili powder

¼ teaspoon sea salt

2½ cups bone broth

2 tablespoons nutritional yeast

½ cup full-fat coconut milk

INSTRUCTIONS

1 Preheat the oven to 400°F.

2 Line the bacon across a baking sheet. Place the pan in the oven and cook for about 20 to 25 minutes or until the bacon is cooked and crispy. Transfer the bacon to a plate lined with a paper towel. Set the bacon aside.

3 Turn your Instant Pot to the Sauté setting. Add the olive oil and onion to the pot and sauté for about 3 minutes. Turn off the Instant Pot.

4 Add the butternut squash, apple, Italian seasoning, spices, broth, and nutritional yeast to the Instant Pot. Secure the lid and select the Pressure Cook/Manual setting. Cook on High pressure for about 10 minutes and then press the Quick-Release button.

5 Heat the coconut milk in a saucepan and transfer the Instant Pot contents to a blender. Blend until smooth. Add the coconut milk to the blender and blend on a low setting to mix.

6 Chop the bacon. Serve soup in a shallow bowl and top with bacon.

Minestrone Soup

A twist on a classic soup. This soup uses lots of vegetables that provide you with vitamins, minerals, and phytonutrients to support your health and avoid inflammation.

INGREDIENTS

2 tablespoons olive oil

1 medium yellow onion, finely diced

2 garlic cloves, minced

1 large carrot, diced

2 stalks celery, diced

1 cup thinly sliced mushrooms

1 medium zucchini, chopped into quarters

1 cup fresh green beans, cut into 2-inch pieces

1 (14.5 oz.) can red kidney beans, drained and rinsed

2 tablespoons tomato paste

1 (15 oz.) can diced tomatoes

8 cups chicken stock or bone broth

Salt and pepper, to taste

1 teaspoon dried oregano

¼ teaspoon Italian seasoning

¼ teaspoon crushed red pepper (optional)

2 cups baby spinach, chopped

1 cup gluten-free pasta of choice, cooked al dente

INSTRUCTIONS

1 Heat the olive oil in a large Dutch oven. Add the onion, garlic, carrot, celery, and mushrooms and sauté for 5 minutes

2 Add the zucchini, green beans, kidney beans, tomato paste, diced tomatoes, broth, salt, pepper, oregano, Italian seasoning, and crushed red pepper.

3 Bring the soup just to a boil and reduce the heat to bring the soup to a simmer. Place the lid on the pot and cook for about 20 to 25 minutes or until the vegetables are tender.

4 Uncover the soup and add the vegetables. Let the soup simmer until the spinach begins to wilt, about 2 to 3 minutes. Add the al dente pasta and serve.

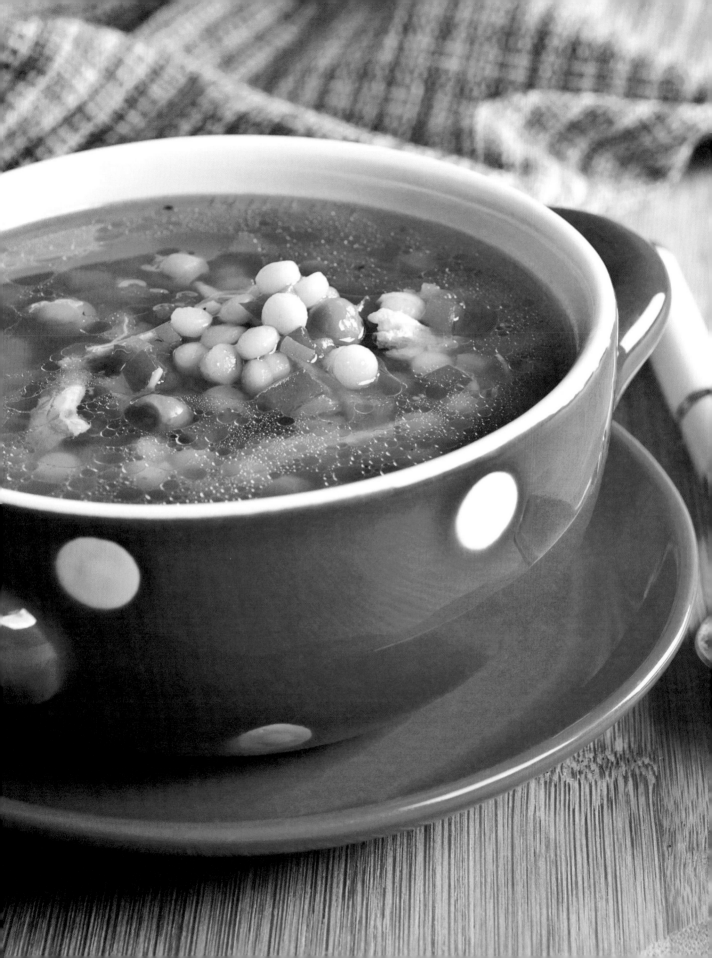

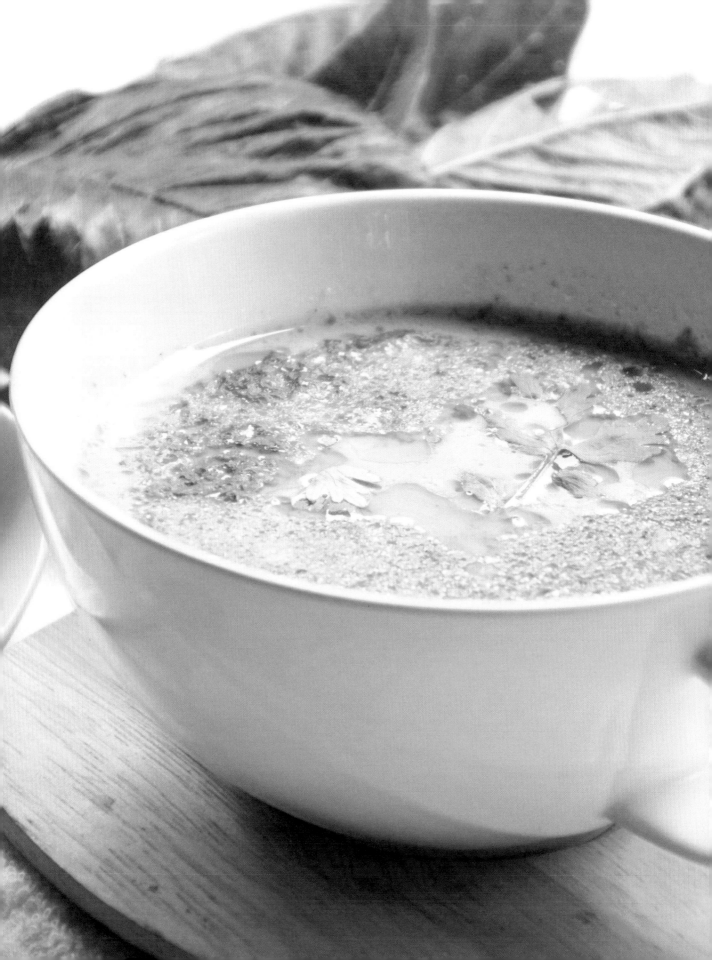

Anti-Inflammatory Broccoli "Cheddar" Soup

There's something so tasty about a broccoli and cheese combo. Here is a version of broccoli cheddar soup that tastes great and uses ingredients to avoid inflammatory responses associated with dairy intake.

INGREDIENTS

2 tablespoons coconut oil

1 small yellow onion, chopped

2 garlic cloves, chopped

1 small head broccoli, stems removed and cut into florets

1 can full-fat coconut milk

1 cup bone broth

⅓ cup raw cashews

1 cup spinach or baby kale

3 tablespoons nutritional yeast

1 teaspoon garlic powder

½ teaspoon onion powder

INSTRUCTIONS

1 In a large Dutch oven, heat the coconut oil and toss in the onion and garlic.

2 Sauté for 3 minutes, add broccoli and sauté for another 4 minutes.

3 Add coconut milk and bone broth and bring to a simmer. Simmer for 8 to 10 minutes.

4 Add the cashews and continue to let simmer for another 7 minutes. Pour the contents of the pot into a high-speed blender along with the spinach, nutritional yeast, garlic powder, and onion powder.

5 Blend until smooth and serve.

Lentil Soup

This hearty soup has everything you need to stay nourished. Lentils are a great source of fiber and protein, as well as zinc, potassium, and magnesium.

INGREDIENTS

2 tablespoons olive oil

1 medium onion, diced

4 garlic cloves, minced

2 medium carrots, chopped

2 celery stalks, diced

1 cup dry lentils, rinsed and sorted

½ teaspoon sea salt

¼ teaspoon black pepper

1 teaspoon dried parsley

½ teaspoon smoked paprika

6 cups bone broth or vegetable stock

⅓ cup chopped scallions, for garnish

INSTRUCTIONS

1   In a large Dutch oven, heat olive oil and add onion and garlic. Sauté for 3 minutes.

2   Add carrots and celery and sauté for 5 minutes. Add lentils and all seasonings. Sauté for 2 minutes.

3   Add the bone broth and bring to a boil. Cover the pot and let the soup simmer for about 25 to 30 minutes. Garnish with the scallions and serve.

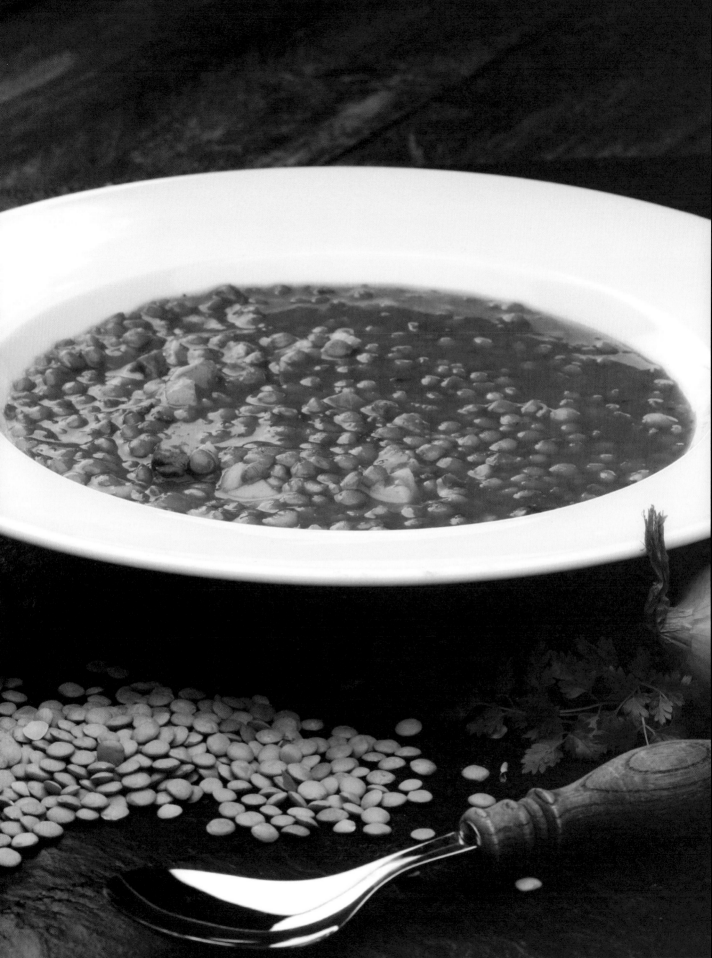

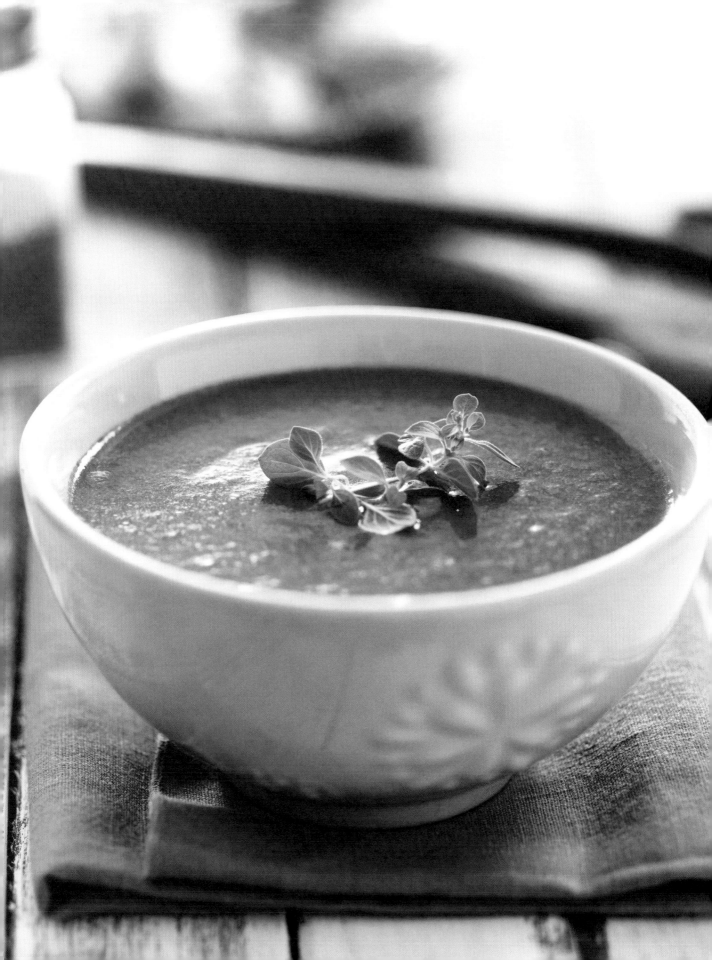

Tomato Bisque

I love a nice tomato soup on a rainy day. Tomatoes have tons of nutrients and phytonutrients that support your immune system. The fat content also helps you feel full and satisfied.

INGREDIENTS

2 tablespoons olive oil

1 small yellow onion, diced

4 garlic cloves, minced

1 (15 oz.) can fire-roasted tomatoes

1 (15 oz.) can crushed tomatoes

1 cup bone broth

Pinch or ⅛ teaspoon crushed red pepper (optional)

1 teaspoon sea salt

½ teaspoon Italian seasoning

½ cup chopped fresh basil

½ cup full-fat coconut milk

INSTRUCTIONS

1 In a large Dutch oven, heat the olive oil and add the onion and garlic. Sauté for 3 to 4 minutes.

2 Add the fire-roasted tomatoes, crushed tomatoes, and bone broth. Season with red pepper flakes, sea salt, and Italian seasoning.

3 Cover the pot and let simmer for about 15 to 20 minutes. Uncover the pot and carefully transfer the soup to a high-speed blender. Add the basil and blend until smooth.

4 Add the coconut milk to the Dutch oven along with the tomato soup. Let the soup simmer for 5 more minutes, then serve.

Immune-Boosting Chicken Soup

This recipe incorporates bone broth, kale, garlic, cumin, mushrooms, and other whole foods that help your immune system function optimally, reduce systemic inflammation, and prevent chronic diseases related to ongoing inflammation.

INGREDIENTS

2 tablespoons olive oil

1 large onion, chopped

3 celery stalks, diced

2 large carrots, diced

1 tablespoon minced garlic

1½ lbs. chicken breast, cubed

12 oz. cremini mushrooms, sliced thin

½ teaspoon dried thyme

½ teaspoon garlic powder

Pinch or ⅛ teaspoon cumin

½ teaspoon Italian seasoning

1½ teaspoons kosher salt

½ teaspoon black pepper

8 cups bone broth

2 bay leaves

¼ teaspoon crushed red pepper (optional)

2 cups chopped kale, stems removed

INSTRUCTIONS

1　Heat the oil in a large Dutch oven over medium heat. Add the onion, celery, carrots, and garlic. Sauté for 3 minutes. Add the chicken and sauté for another 5 minutes.

2　Add the mushrooms along with the thyme, garlic powder, cumin, Italian seasoning, salt, and pepper. Add in the bone broth, bay leaves, and crushed red pepper, if using. Bring to a simmer, cover, and cook for 15 to 20 minutes or until chicken is cooked through.

3　Uncover and stir in the kale. Put the lid back on and cook for another 5 to 7 minutes or until the kale is tender.

4　Adjust the seasoning as needed and serve.

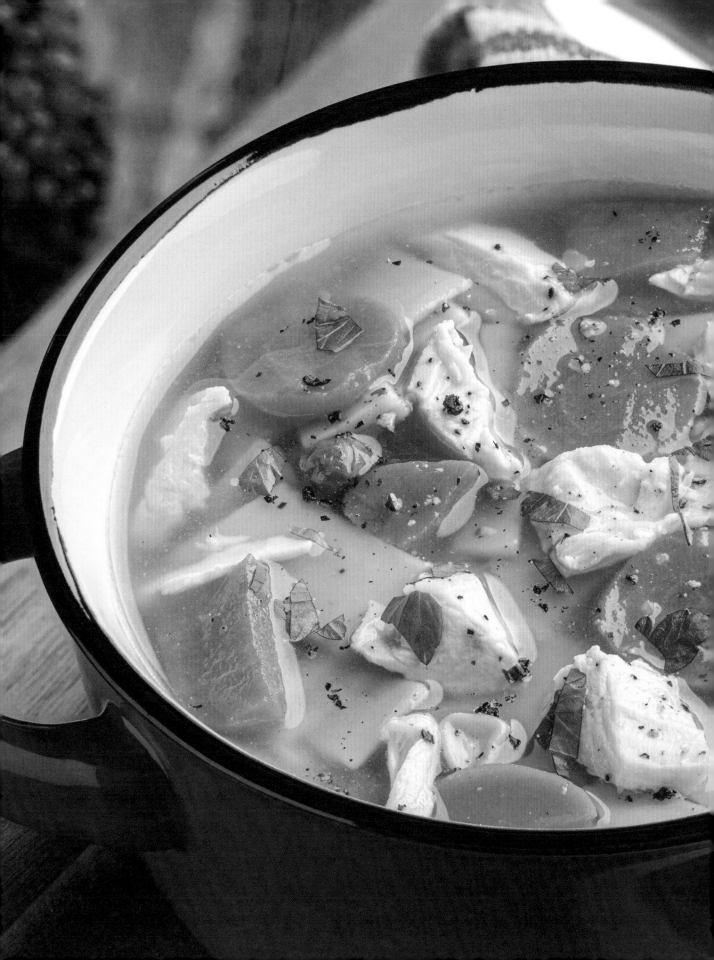

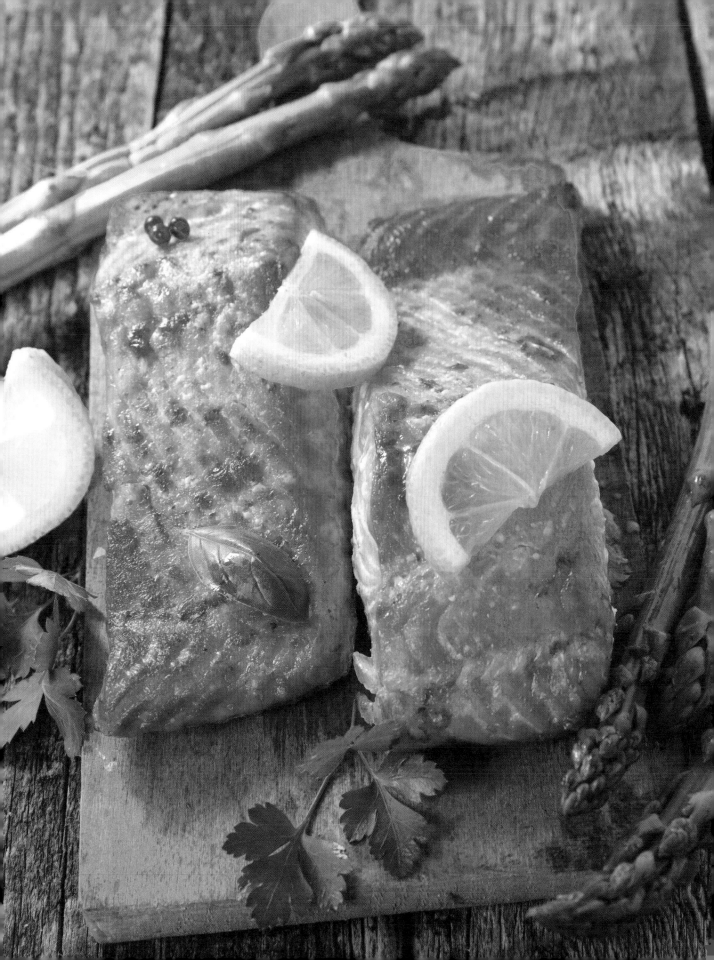

One-Pan Salmon & Asparagus Bake

Looking for a quick dinner with minimal cleanup? This one-pan dish is
perfect for a quick fix meal without compromising nutrition.

INGREDIENTS

4 tablespoons extra-virgin
olive oil

2 tablespoons fresh lemon juice

4 garlic cloves, finely minced

1 tablespoon fresh dill

½ teaspoon sea salt

¼ teaspoon black pepper

1¼ lbs. wild-caught salmon,
cut into 4 portions (you may
also use 4 pre-cut frozen
wild-caught salmon filets)

1 lb. or 1 bunch asparagus,
rinsed and ends cut

½ small red onion, thinly sliced

½ lemon, thinly sliced

INSTRUCTIONS

1 Preheat oven to 425°F.

2 Line a large rimmed baking sheet with parchment paper.

3 Whisk together the oil, lemon juice, garlic, dill, sea salt,
   and pepper to create a marinade.

4 Place the salmon fillets on the parchment paper along the
   center of the pan.

5 Arrange trimmed asparagus and onion on the sides of the
   salmon.

6 Pour the marinade over the salmon and asparagus.

7 Use a pair of tongs (or clean hands) to toss the asparagus
   and rub marinade over the salmon.

8 Top each salmon with a thin slice of lemon.

9 Place pan in the oven and bake for 15 to 20 minutes.
   Check salmon for doneness. If it flakes easily with a fork
   and is no longer dark or opaque, it's done.

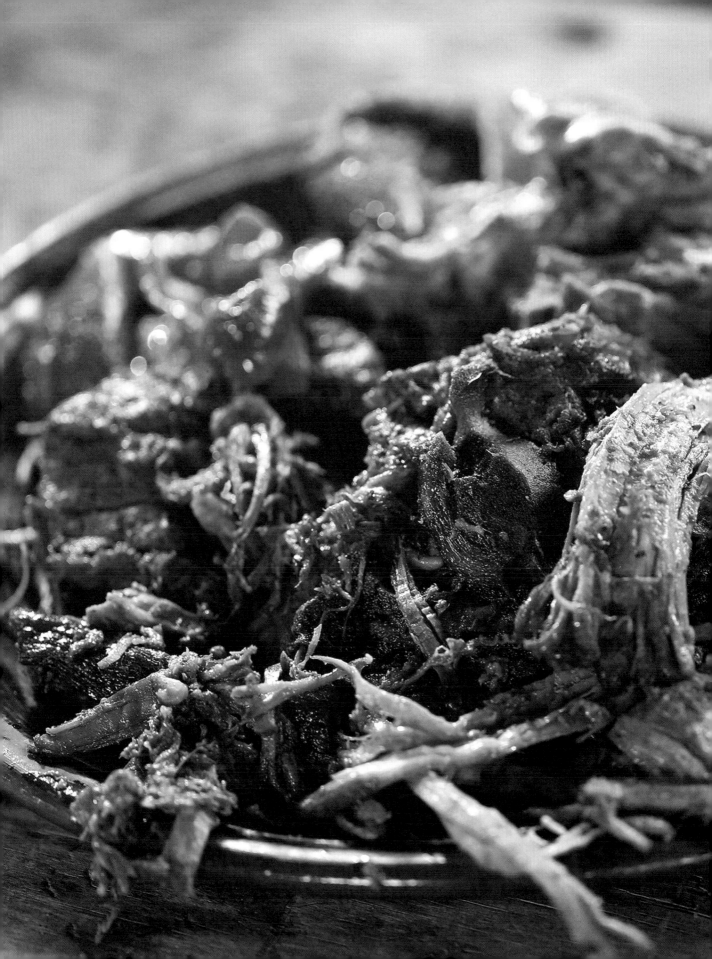

Easy Pork Carnitas

Need something easy but tasty for dinner? No need to reach for the take-out menu! This recipe uses an Instant Pot or pressure cooker so you can enjoy tender, high-quality protein with ease.

INGREDIENTS

2 teaspoons sea salt

1 teaspoon black pepper

1 teaspoon onion powder

1 teaspoon garlic powder

½ teaspoon cumin

1 teaspoon dried oregano

3-4 lbs. pork loin, boneless

1 (15 oz.) can fire-roasted tomatoes

INSTRUCTIONS

1   Add all of the dry ingredients to a small bowl and whisk together.

2   Place the pork into an Instant Pot or pressure cooker. Rub the seasoning mixture all over the pork.

3   Add the can of fire-roasted tomatoes.

4   Secure the lid and select Pressure Cook/Manual on High pressure for about 40 minutes.

5   Let pressure release naturally for about 20 minutes or until the pin drops.

6   Remove the pork to a large bowl and shred with two forks.

7   Serve the pork with your favorite tortilla, side salad, or brown rice.

Apple & Chicken Curry

Not only is this recipe delicious, but it also uses curry, which is packed with anti-inflammatory nutrients like curcumin. Serve this curry over rice, cauliflower rice, your favorite salad greens, or eat it alone for a warm and satisfying meal.

INGREDIENTS

2 teaspoons olive oil, avocado oil, or coconut oil

1 medium yellow onion, diced

4 garlic cloves, minced

1 large apple, peeled and cubed

1 ½ lbs. chicken breast, cubed

Sea salt, to taste, plus ½ teaspoon

Cayenne pepper, to taste, plus ¼ teaspoon

⅔ cup chicken broth

3 tablespoon curry powder

Continued...

INSTRUCTIONS

1   In a large skillet on medium-high heat, add your cooking oil of choice. Once hot, add the onion, garlic, and apple.

2   Sauté for about 5 to 7 minutes or until apples are slightly tender. Remove the mixture from heat.

3   Add the chicken to the pan and sprinkle with a pinch of salt and pepper. Let the chicken cook for about 12 to 15 minutes or until golden brown. Remove the chicken from the pan.

4   Add the chicken broth, curry powder, cumin, turmeric, ½ teaspoon sea salt, garlic powder, ¼ teaspoon cayenne pepper, and coconut milk to the pan. Whisk until the ingredients are well combined.

5   Let the sauce mixture simmer in the pan for about 10 minutes or until it thickens.

6   Once the sauce thickens, add the chicken back into the pan, along with the onion-apple mixture.

7   Add in the spinach and toss until the spinach softens, about 3 to 5 minutes. Garnish with the cilantro and serve.

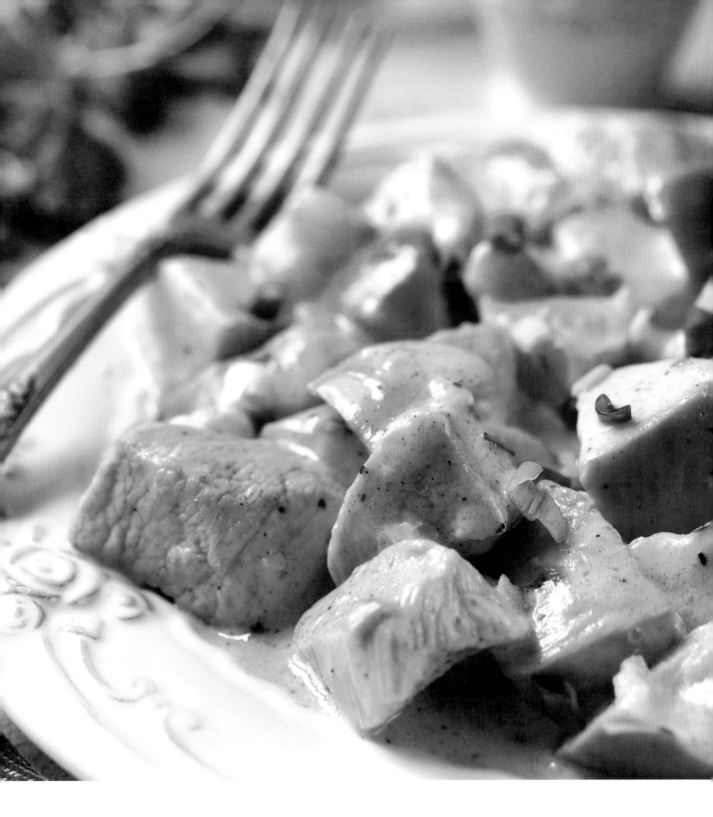

| 2 teaspoons ground cumin | ¼ teaspoon garlic powder | 2 cups spinach, chopped |
| 1 teaspoon ground turmeric | 1 can (14 oz.) full-fat coconut milk | ¼ cup cilantro, roughly chopped, for garnish |

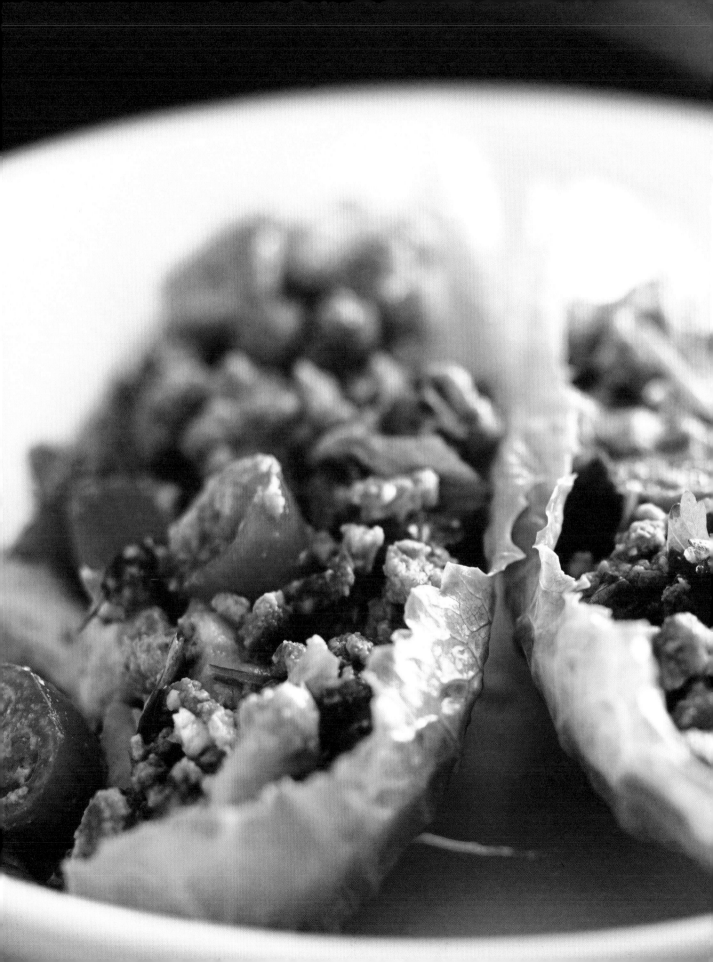

Lettuce Wrap Tacos

This is a great twist to your regular taco. Using a lettuce wrap is a great substitute for a taco wrap because it adds extra crunch and tons of nutrients like vitamin A, vitamin K, and folate, while avoiding inflammatory responses that may arise when eating a flour tortilla.

INGREDIENTS

3 tablespoons avocado oil

1 medium onion, minced

3 garlic cloves, minced

1 lb. ground turkey

¼ teaspoon sea salt

2 tablespoons Taco Seasoning (see recipe on page 97)

1 tablespoon nutritional yeast

2 cups baby spinach or baby kale leaves, chopped

1 can black beans, rinsed and drained

6 butter leaf lettuce cups or romaine lettuce cups, cleaned and dry

1 Hass avocado, sliced, for serving or guacamole (optional)

Homemade Salsa, for serving (optional, see recipe on page 102)

INSTRUCTIONS

1 In a medium skillet, heat the oil and add the onion and garlic. Sauté for about 5 to 6 minutes or until the onions become translucent and fragrant.

2 Add the turkey, salt, Taco Seasoning, and nutritional yeast and mix while continuing to break down the turkey chunks with a spatula. Cook until the turkey is cooked through, about 10 to 15 minutes.

3 Add the spinach and cook until wilted, about 2 minutes. Turn the heat to low and add the beans.

4 Mash the beans until smooth using a fork.

5 Remove the beans from the heat and spoon the turkey into the lettuce cups.

6 Top with avocado or salsa, if desired.

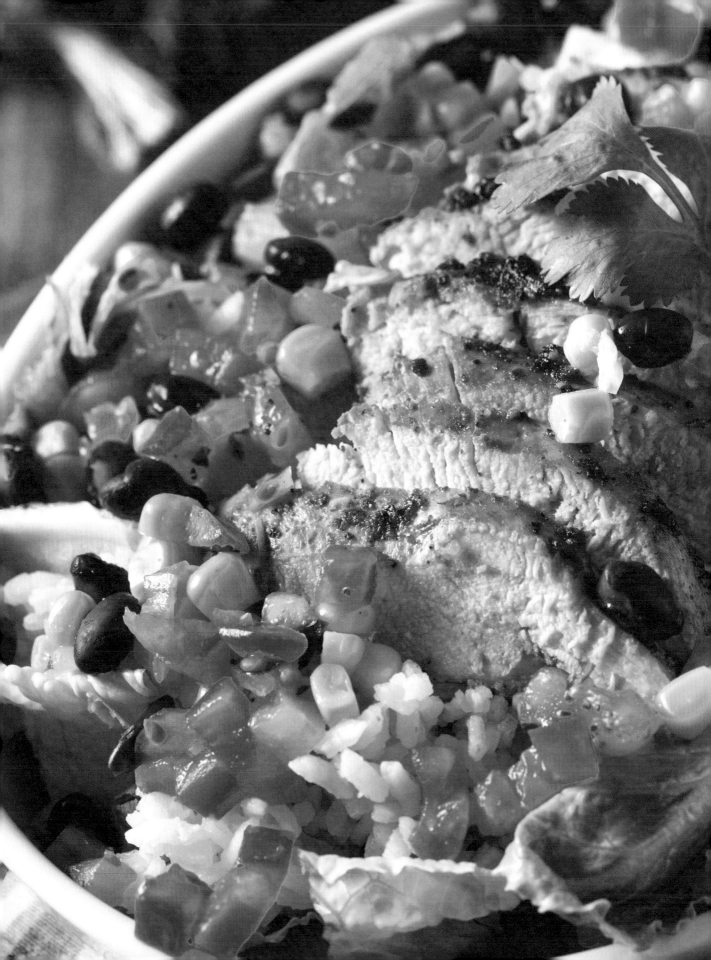

Homemade Burrito Bowl

Here is a recipe that will keep you moving towards your nutritional goals regardless of how short you are on time. You can use leftover chicken or buy an organic rotisserie chicken from the store. The vegetables also keep this meal packed with anti-inflammatory nutrients without taking up too much time.

INGREDIENTS

16 oz. leftover chicken or store-bought rotisserie chicken, shredded

3 cups mixed salad greens

½ small red onion, thinly sliced

1 tablespoon lime juice

1 tablespoon extra-virgin olive oil

¼ teaspoon sea salt

Pinch of black pepper

4 cups white or brown rice, cooked

½ cup Homemade Salsa (see recipe on page 102)

1 Hass avocado, sliced

¼ cup cilantro, chopped, for garnish

INSTRUCTIONS

1   Heat leftover chicken as desired.

2   In a medium-size mixing bowl, add greens, onion, lime juice, olive oil, salt, and pepper. Mix well using tongs.

3   Divide greens into serving bowls and top with rice.

4   Place chicken on top of rice and top with Homemade Salsa and avocado. Garnish with cilantro.

Optional: Dress the mixed salad with 2-3 tablespoons of Cilantro-Lime Vinaigrette (see recipe on page 93).

Instant Pot Lemon Chicken with Asparagus

This is a simple meal that's packed with amazing flavor and is rich in antioxidants that support your immune system, increase liver detoxification, and avoid chronic inflammation from waste and toxin build-up.

INGREDIENTS

1 tablespoon Italian seasoning

2 tablespoons lemon zest

1 teaspoon sea salt

½ teaspoon black pepper

½ teaspoon garlic powder

½ teaspoon onion powder

¼ teaspoon smoked paprika

4-6 boneless chicken thighs

3 tablespoons olive oil

3-4 garlic cloves, minced

1 cup water

Juice of 1 lemon

1 bunch asparagus, fibrous ends cut off

2 tablespoons chopped roasted pistachios or pine nuts, for garnish

INSTRUCTIONS

1 Preheat oven to 375°F.

2 In a small bowl, combine the Italian seasoning, lemon zest, and spices and mix with a fork. Pat the chicken thighs dry with a paper towel and season with the dry seasoning mixture, as desired.

3 Turn the Instant Pot to the Sauté setting and add 2 tablespoons olive oil. Once hot, place the garlic and chicken thighs in the pot.

Continued...

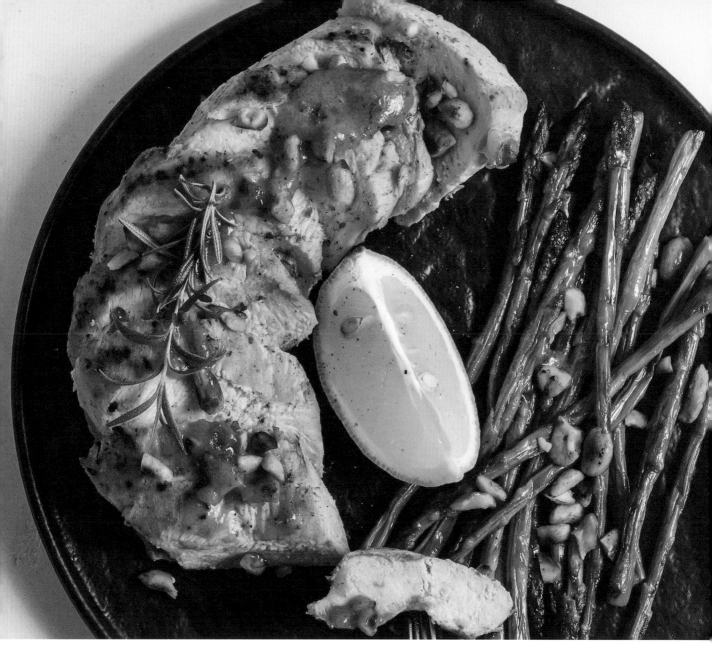

4 Let the chicken cook for about 3 to 4 minutes and then flip it over. Cook for another 3 minutes. Remove the chicken from the Instant Pot and turn it off.

5 Pour in 1 cup of water and place the metal rack inside of the Instant Pot. Place the chicken thighs on top of the rack and pour lemon juice over the chicken. Cover the Instant Pot with a lid and set it to Pressure Cook/Manual on High for about 8 to 10 minutes.

6 While the chicken cooks, place the asparagus on a sheet pan. Drizzle with the remaining olive oil and salt and pepper to taste. Mix in the seasoning and place in the oven for about 12 to 15 minutes.

7 Once the pressure cooker finishes cooking, allow the chicken to natural release for 5 minutes then press the Quick-Release button. Remove chicken from pot and serve with asparagus and nuts.

Chicken & Broccoli Stir-Fry

This is a great substitute for your average stir-fry from your local take-out spot. Without compromising great taste, this recipe avoids inflammatory ingredients (including MSG) and uses anti-inflammatory ingredients like ginger, garlic, coconut aminos, and broccoli. This recipe also swaps out cornstarch for arrowroot powder, which is a great thickener for sauces, slurries, or gravies.

INGREDIENTS

1½-2 lbs. chicken breasts, sliced and cubed

2 tablespoons coconut aminos

3 tablespoons avocado oil, plus 1 tablespoon

2 teaspoons rice wine vinegar

¼ teaspoon black pepper

¼ teaspoon garlic powder

½ teaspoon sea salt

Pinch of crushed red pepper (optional)

3 cups broccoli florets

1-2 tablespoons water

¼ cup scallions, chopped (optional, for garnish)

Continued...

INSTRUCTIONS

1 In a large mixing bowl, combine the cubed chicken breast, coconut aminos, 3 tablespoons avocado oil, rice wine vinegar, pepper, garlic powder, sea salt, and crushed red pepper, if using. Cover and put in the fridge for at least 30 minutes before cooking.

2 In a smaller bowl, put all the sauce ingredients together and whisk until well combined.

3 In a large skillet, heat 1 tablespoon avocado oil. Place chicken in the pan and sauté for about 10 to 13 minutes or until the chicken becomes golden brown. Remove chicken from the pan

4 Place broccoli florets in the pan and pour in 1-2 tablespoons water. Move broccoli around and cover. Cook broccoli for about 3 minutes.

5 Uncover pan and let broccoli cook for another minute, then add the chicken back. Add in sauce and continue to sauté until the sauce begins to thicken.

6 Garnish with the scallions. Eat alone or serve with rice.

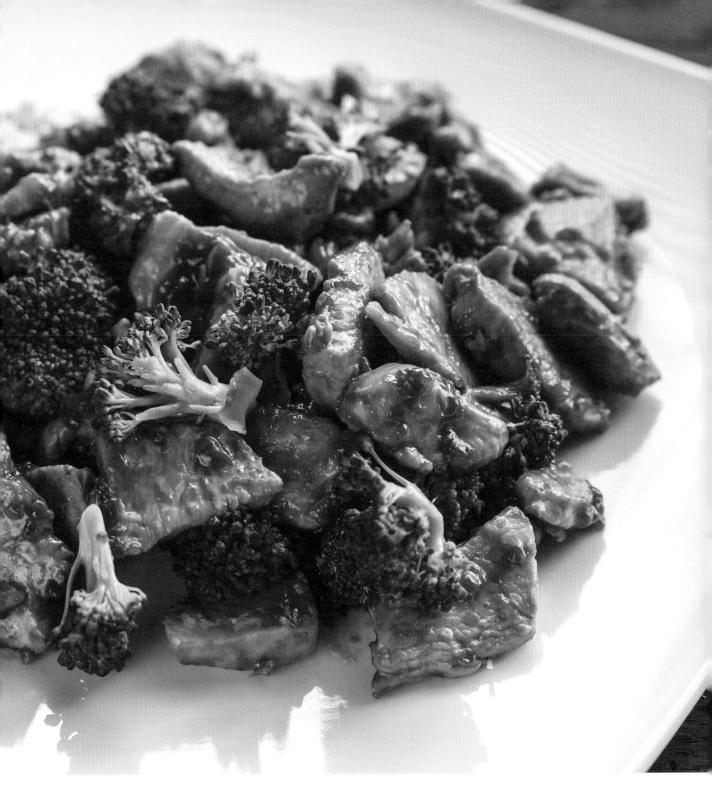

Sauce

¼ cup coconut aminos

1 teaspoon toasted sesame oil

1 teaspoon toasted sesame seeds

½ teaspoon sea salt

¼ teaspoon minced ginger

¼ cup chicken broth

2 teaspoons arrowroot powder

Creamy Italian Chicken

This is a great Sunday dinner. This recipe calls for coconut milk instead of heavy cream as most people are sensitive to dairy without even knowing it. People who continue to eat foods they are sensitive to (even if they don't know they're sensitive) will continue to trigger an inflammatory response within their bodies.

INGREDIENTS

3 tablespoons grass-fed butter, ghee, or avocado oil

1½ lbs. boneless skinless chicken breasts, sliced thin

Salt and pepper, to taste

¼ teaspoon garlic powder

2 cups dinosaur kale, chopped

1 medium onion, diced

6 garlic cloves, minced

Pinch or ⅛ teaspoon crushed red pepper (optional)

1 cup coconut milk or your choice of creamy milk (can use heavy cream for keto)

Continued...

INSTRUCTIONS

1 Heat 2 tablespoons cooking fat in a large skillet over medium-high heat and season chicken with salt, pepper, and garlic powder.

2 Place chicken in the pan and cook for 5 to 6 minutes on each side. Remove chicken from pan.

3 Add the last 1 tablespoon of cooking fat to the pan and heat. Add the kale, onion, garlic, and crushed red pepper, if using. Season with the salt and pepper to taste.

4 Sauté the vegetables for about 4 minutes or until kale starts to become tender. Remove from pan.

5 Add coconut milk, broth, and lemon juice and stir. Continue scraping the bottom of the pan to deglaze. Bring to a boil then reduce heat to a simmer. Let simmer for about 6 to 7 minutes or until sauce begins to thicken.

6 Add the chicken and vegetables. Add the sun-dried tomatoes and basil. Cook for another 3 to 4 minutes. Garnish with Parmesan cheese, if using, and serve.

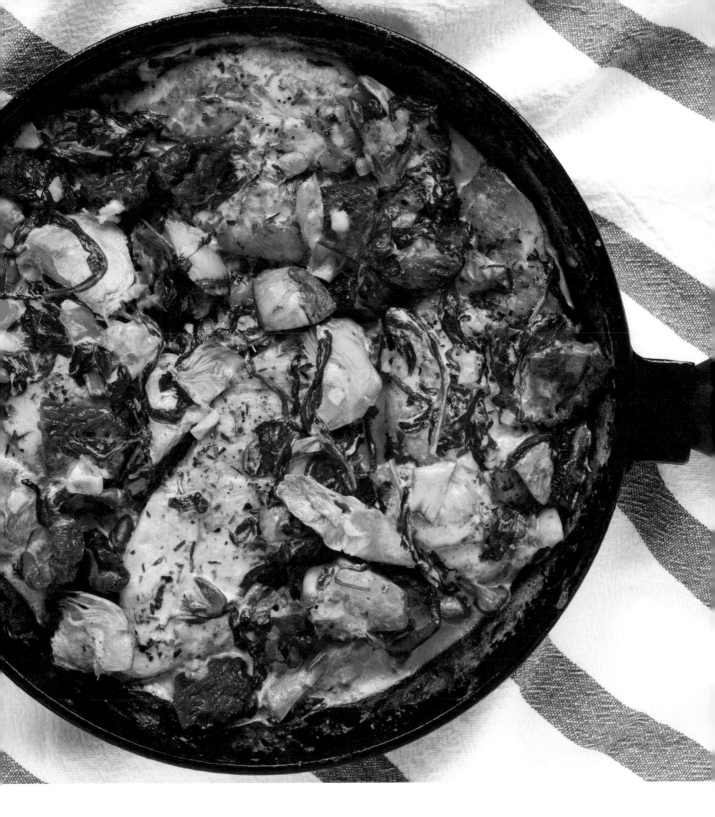

½ cup chicken broth

Juice of 1 lemon

½ cup sun-dried tomatoes, chopped

1 cup basil leaves, julienned

Parmesan cheese, for garnish (optional, omit if sensitive to dairy)

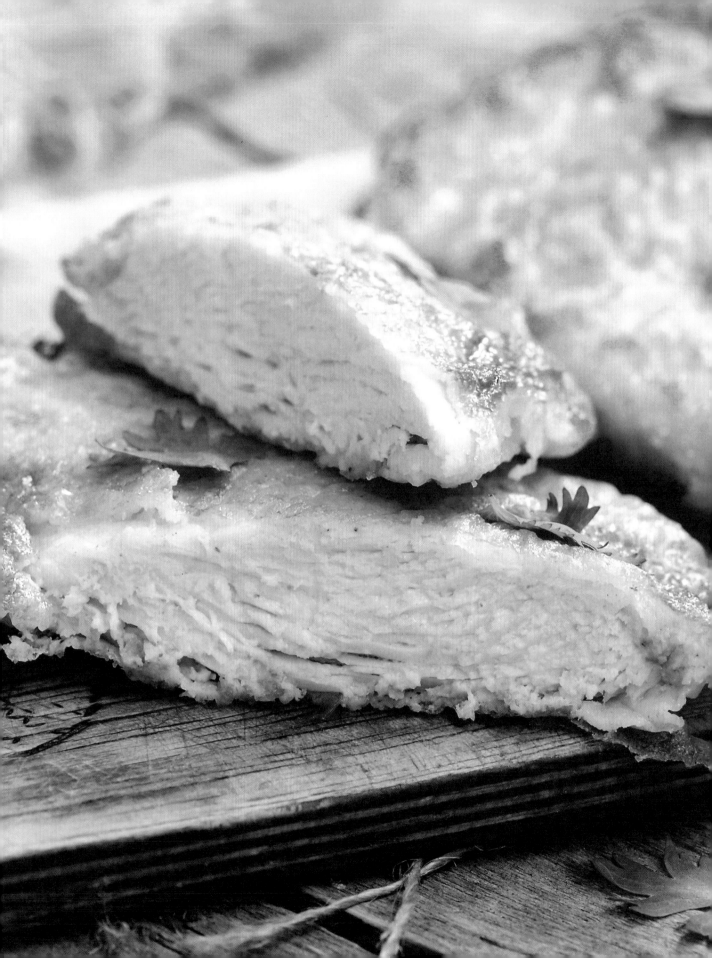

"Fried" Chicken Cutlets

The ultimate comfort food. My husband grew up eating fried chicken cutlets in his Italian household and these cutlets always remind him of "the good 'ol days." Once we started living together, I had to learn how to make this comfort food without the inflammatory ingredients and cooking oils.

INGREDIENTS

1½-2 lbs. chicken breast, sliced thin

2 whole pasture-raised eggs, beaten

⅓ cup non-dairy milk

2 cups almond flour or meal

1 tablespoon garlic powder

½ tablespoon onion powder

1 teaspoon paprika

2 teaspoons salt

1 teaspoon black pepper

1 tablespoon Italian seasoning

¼ teaspoon baking powder

Coconut cooking spray

INSTRUCTIONS

1 Preheat the air fryer to 400°F.

2 Pat the chicken tenders dry with a paper towel and set them aside.

3 In one bowl, add the eggs and non-dairy milk and whisk until well combined.

4 In another shallow bowl, combine the almond flour or meal, spices, Italian seasoning, and baking powder and mix until well combined.

5 Dip each chicken cutlet into the egg mixture first and then coat well with the dry mixture.

6 Spray the bottom of the air fryer basket and the tops of the chicken cutlets with cooking spray and place the chicken cutlets in the fryer.

7 Cook in the air fryer for about 12 to 14 minutes, stopping the timer halfway to flip the cutlets.

8 Spray the other side of the cutlets with cooking spray. Continue until all cutlets are cooked.

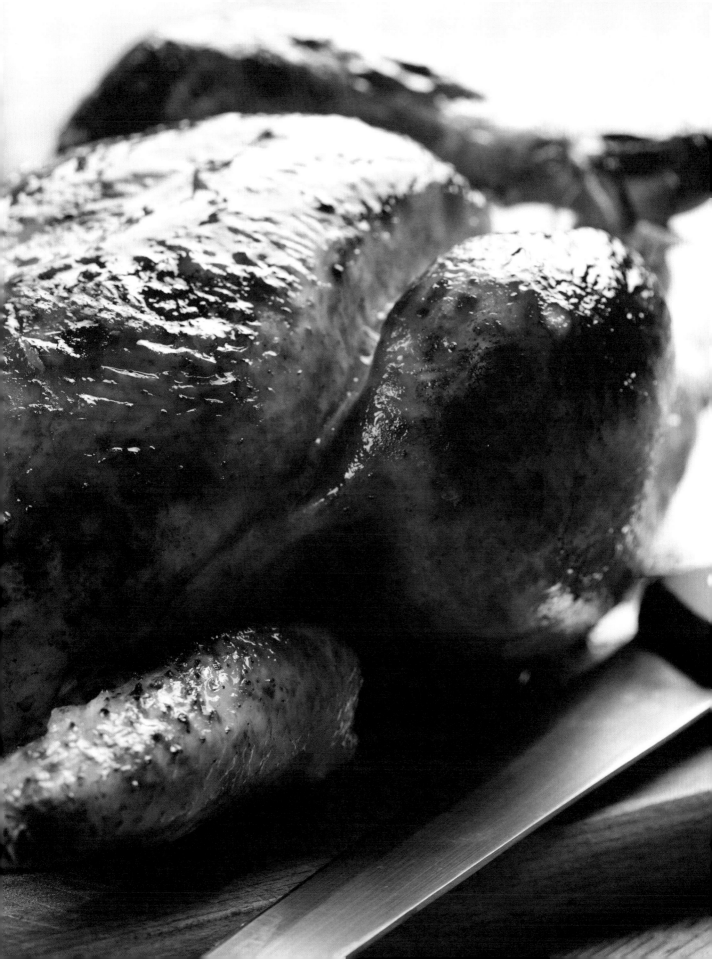

Roasted Chicken

Not only does this simple and delicious recipe use herbs with anti-inflammatory properties, it's also great for meal prepping. This roasted chicken pairs perfectly with any side or vegetable, and its leftovers can be used to prepare salads and soups to keep your health goals on track.

INGREDIENTS

3½ lbs. whole chicken

½ tablespoon salt

½ tablespoon garlic powder

½ tablespoon dried oregano

1 teaspoon onion powder

1 teaspoon cumin

¼ teaspoon black pepper

½ teaspoon turmeric

INSTRUCTIONS

1   Preheat the oven to 375°F.

2   Rinse the chicken well and remove the giblet bag. Dry the chicken very well with a paper towel and set it aside.

3   In a small mixing bowl, mix all of the seasonings.

4   Gradually pour or use your fingers to coat chicken with the dry seasoning mixture. Be sure to use your fingers to get underneath the chicken skin to season the breast and leg meat.

5   Place chicken in a baking dish or a cast-iron skillet and bake uncovered at 375°F for about 1 hour and 15 minutes to 1 hour and 30 minutes, or until an internal temperature of 165°F is reached.

One-Pan Chicken & Vegetables

This is a simple recipe with very little cleanup required, but it's packed with many antioxidants and phytonutrients that will help fight inflammation and make sure you're feeling your best.

INGREDIENTS

Cooking spray

1½ lbs. boneless skinless chicken thighs

½ teaspoon kosher salt, divided

¼ teaspoon black pepper

2 tablespoons extra-virgin olive oil, divided

1 small head broccoli, cut into medium-sized florets

1 small head cauliflower, cut into medium-sized florets

1 red bell pepper, cored and sliced

1 zucchini, chopped

1 medium red onion, sliced

Continued...

INSTRUCTIONS

1 Preheat the oven to 400°F and coat a sheet pan with cooking spray.

2 Place the chicken thighs on the pan and season with salt and pepper and drizzle with 1 tablespoon olive oil.

3 In a large mixing bowl, add the broccoli, cauliflower, red bell pepper, zucchini, and onion. Season the vegetables with 1 tablespoon olive oil, lemon juice, lemon zest, Italian seasoning, garlic powder, onion powder, salt and pepper to taste, and nutritional yeast.

4 Place the vegetables on the tray surrounding the chicken. Place in the oven and bake for about 25 to 27 minutes or until the chicken has reached an internal temperature of 165°F.

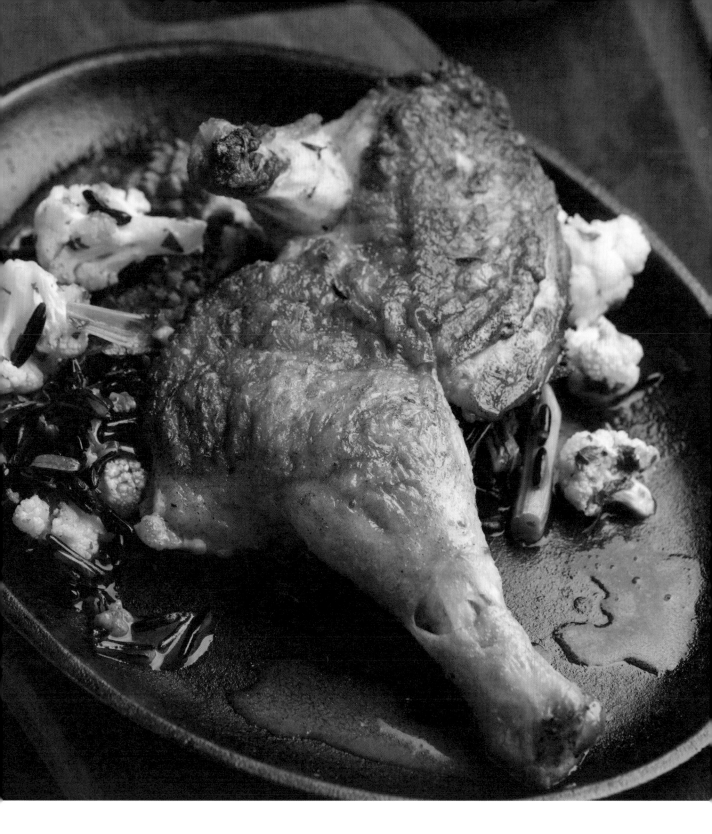

| 1 tablespoon lemon juice | 1 teaspoon Italian seasoning | 1 teaspoon onion powder |
| ½ teaspoon lemon zest | 1 teaspoon garlic powder | 1 tablespoon nutritional yeast |

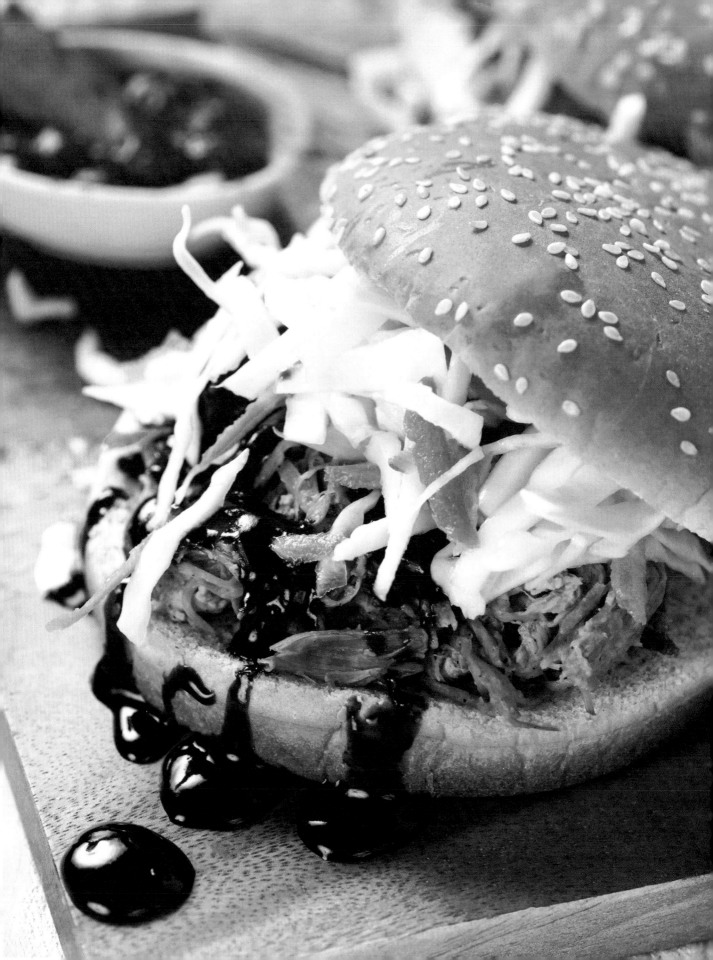

Instant Pot Pulled BBQ Chicken with Sweet Potato Fries

Yes, you can enjoy BBQ chicken while eating an anti-inflammatory diet. The key is to read the ingredients on the BBQ sauce label and opt for one that is not loaded with sugar and partially hydrogenated oils. I like to use the Primal Kitchen BBQ sauce.

INGREDIENTS

3 boneless skinless chicken breasts

Salt and pepper, to taste

½ teaspoon garlic powder

½ teaspoon onion powder

1 cup Whole30 BBQ sauce

Cooking spray

2 medium-sized sweet potatoes, sliced into ¼-inch slices

1 tablespoon olive oil

¼ teaspoon cinnamon

INSTRUCTIONS

1 Preheat the oven to 400°F.

2 Season the chicken with salt, pepper, garlic powder, and onion powder and place it in the Instant Pot.

3 Pour the BBQ sauce all over the chicken, close the lid, and set the timer on the pressure cooker to 15 minutes.

4 Coat a sheet pan with cooking spray. In a mixing bowl, mix sweet potatoes, olive oil, salt, and cinnamon. Toss to combine and cover sweet potatoes in seasoning.

5 Line baking sheet with sweet potatoes and place in the oven for 20 to 25 minutes. Flip the potatoes halfway through.

6 Let pressure release naturally for about 5 minutes and then press the Quick-Release button. Shred the chicken with two forks. Serve alone or with coleslaw and gluten-free buns, if desired.

Quick Bruschetta Grilled Chicken

This dish is delicious, refreshing, and packed with lycopene, an anti-inflammatory carotenoid that helps calm immune responses when triggered.

INGREDIENTS

2 tablespoons extra-virgin olive oil, plus 3 teaspoons

1½ lbs. boneless skinless chicken breasts, sliced thin

1 cup diced fresh tomatoes

¼ cup diced cucumbers

¼ cup diced red onions

2 tablespoons chopped fresh basil leaves

Salt and pepper, to taste

¼ cup balsamic vinegar

INSTRUCTIONS

1 Heat 2 tablespoons olive oil in a large skillet. Add the chicken and cook for about 6 minutes on each side or until the inside is no longer pink.

2 In a mixing bowl, add the tomatoes, cucumber, and onion. Top the mixture with basil, salt and pepper to taste, 3 teaspoons olive oil, and balsamic vinegar. Mix well to combine.

3 Once it's done cooking, let the chicken cool on a plate and top with bruschetta.

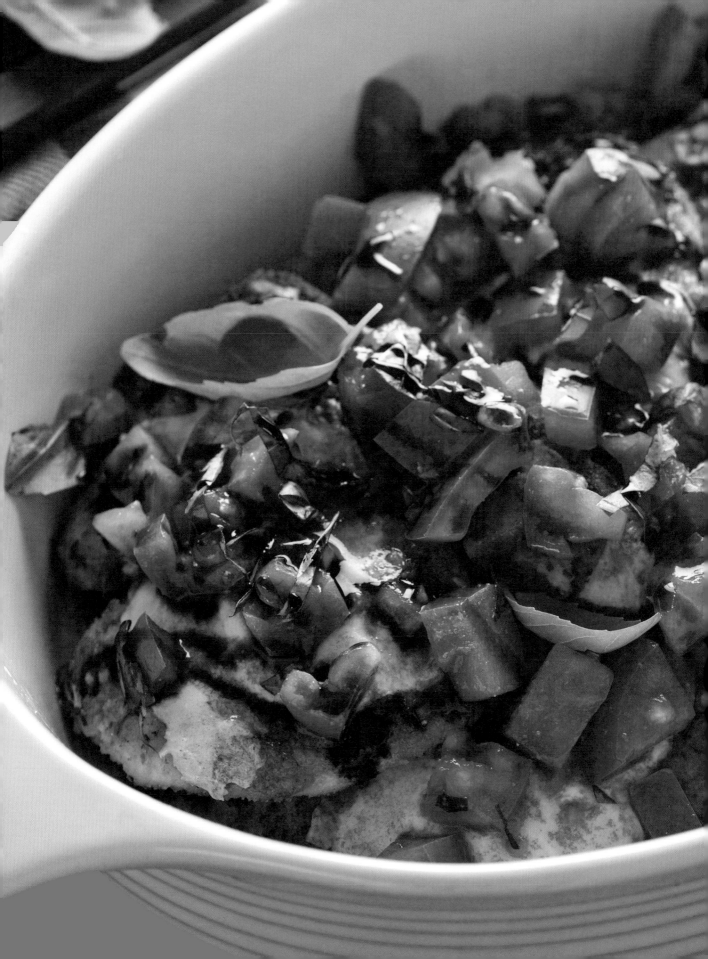

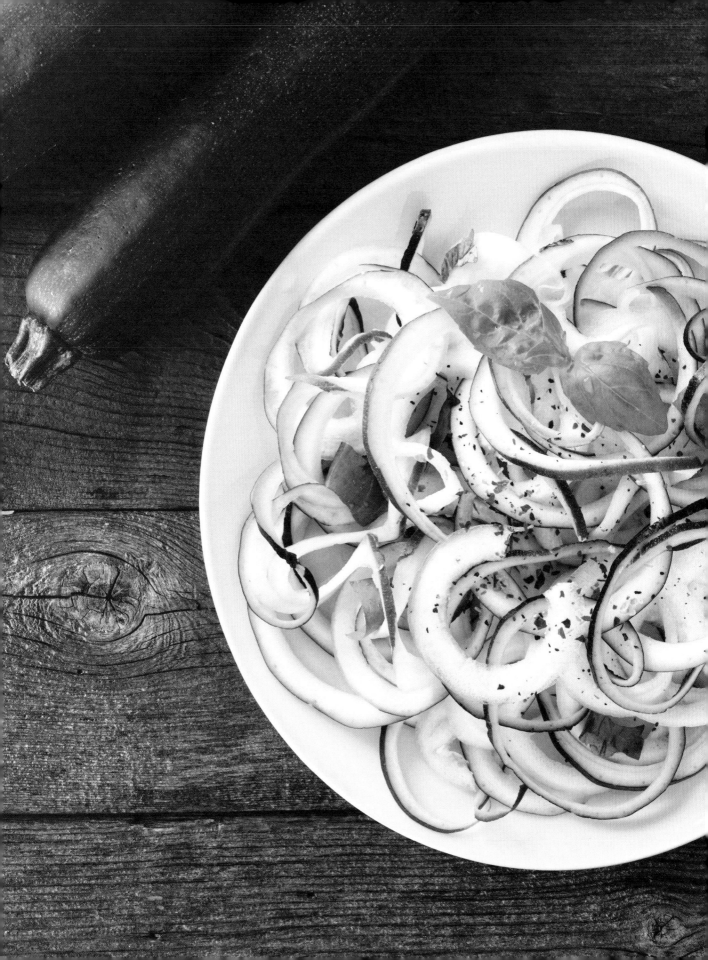

Buttery Garlic Zucchini Noodles

Zucchini noodles are a great option if you're not using a traditional marinara sauce. In my opinion, zucchini noodles taste best with a lighter sauce. If you're sensitive to dairy, use ghee instead of butter. Both grass-fed ghee and butter are known to be higher in anti-inflammatory omega-3 fatty acids.

INGREDIENTS

3 tablespoons salted butter or ghee

6 garlic cloves, minced

¼ cup minced yellow onion

2-3 medium zucchinis, spiraled

Salt and pepper, to taste

¼ cup minced fresh parsley

1 teaspoon lemon zest

INSTRUCTIONS

1   Melt the butter in a large skillet over medium heat. Add the minced garlic and onion and sauté until garlic becomes fragrant, about 1 to 2 minutes.

2   Stir in the zucchini noodles and cook until the noodles just become tender, about 2 to 3 minutes. Do not overcook noodles or they will become soggy and easily breakable. Season with salt and pepper to taste.

3   Remove the noodles from the heat and toss in the parsley and lemon zest, then serve.

Pesto Salmon with Asparagus

This is a quick and easy nutrient-rich meal. There's plenty of quality protein, fat, and fiber to keep you feeling full and satisfied.

INGREDIENTS

3 tablespoons avocado oil, divided

1 bunch asparagus, fibrous ends trimmed off

1 tablespoon lemon juice

Sea salt and black pepper, to taste

2 tablespoons chopped roasted pistachios or pine nuts

4 (3 oz.) fillets wild-caught salmon

1 cup Packed Pesto (see recipe on page 98)

⅓ cup chopped scallions, for garnish

INSTRUCTIONS

1   In a large skillet, heat 1 tablespoon avocado oil. Add the asparagus and sauté for 5 minutes. Add the lemon juice, salt and pepper to taste, and nuts.

2   Cook for another 5 minutes and then remove the asparagus from the pan.

3   Add 2 more tablespoons avocado oil to the pan. Once hot, add the salmon filets and season with salt and pepper to taste. Cook for about 3 to 5 minutes on each side.

4   Remove the filets from the pan and top with the pistachios and a heaping spoon of Pesto. Spread the Pesto over the salmon and garnish with scallions.

5   Serve the Pesto salmon with the asparagus, and garnish with the scallions.

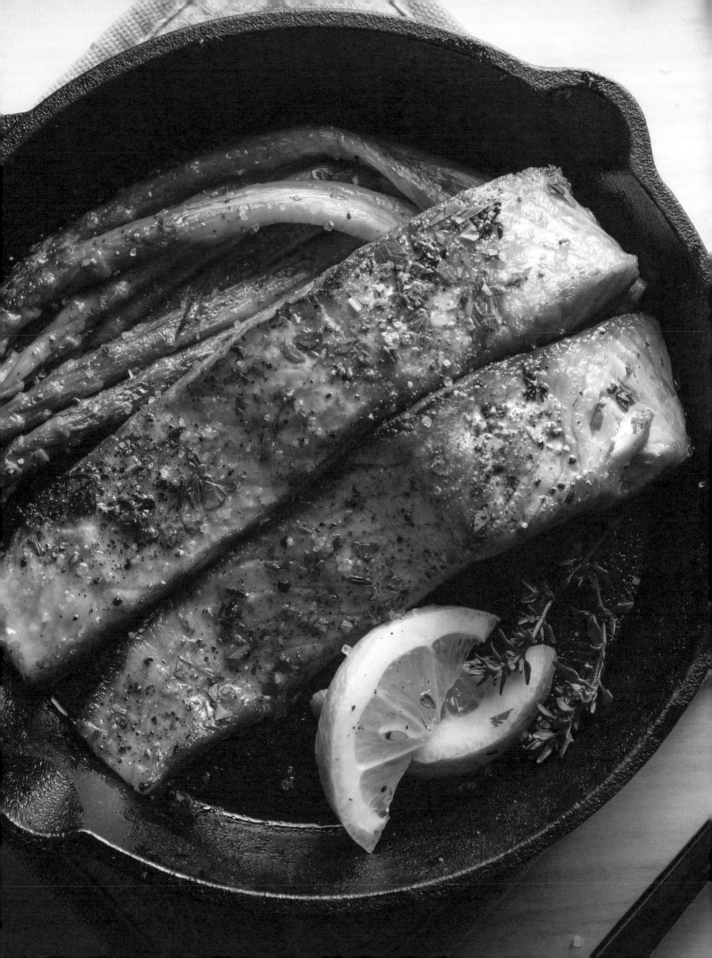

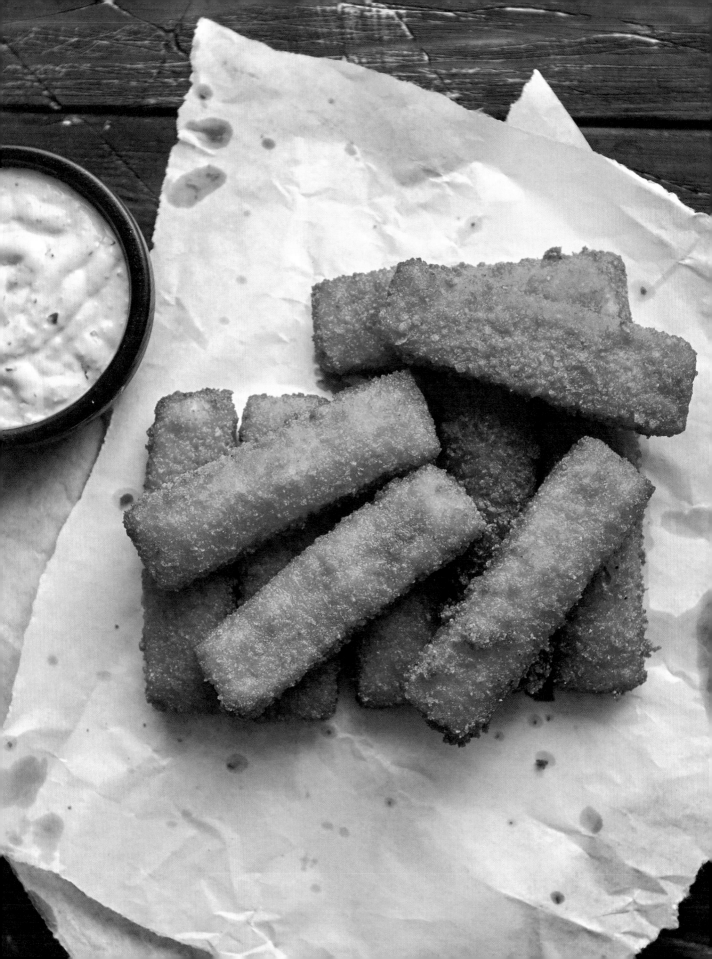

Fish Sticks

A childhood favorite that can be eaten at any age. This recipe uses wild-caught fish and almond flour instead of regular flour to avoid triggering inflammation within your body. Enjoy with a side of your favorite vegetables.

INGREDIENTS

Olive oil or avocado oil cooking spray

2 whole pasture-raised eggs, whisked very well

1 cup almond flour

1 teaspoon garlic powder

1 teaspoon onion powder

1 teaspoon sweet or smoked paprika

1 teaspoon salt

½ teaspoon dried parsley

½ teaspoon black pepper

1 lb. cod fillets, cut into ½ inch thick slices

INSTRUCTIONS

1 Preheat the oven to 425°F.

2 Spray a baking sheet with cooking spray. Whisk the eggs in one bowl. In another bowl, stir the flour and spices until combined.

3 Using one slice of fish at a time, coat the cod in egg and then cover in dry ingredients. Place on a baking sheet. Repeat until all the fish sticks are coated in the dry mixture.

4 Spray the fish sticks with cooking spray and bake in the oven for about 16 minutes. Turn the fish sticks over at the halfway point and spray again with cooking spray.

Grilled Salmon Taco Bowl with Avocado Salsa

A great addition to your Taco Tuesday festivities. Wild-caught salmon is an excellent source of selenium and omega-3 fatty acids, which are essential for proper immune health. Avocado provides omega-3 fatty acids and fiber.

INGREDIENTS

½ teaspoon cumin

½ teaspoon lime zest

½ teaspoon chili powder

½ teaspoon salt

¼ teaspoon black pepper

4 (3 oz.) wild-caught salmon filets

2 tablespoons avocado oil

4 cups cooked white, brown, or cauliflower rice

Continued...

INSTRUCTIONS

1 In a small bowl, combine the cumin, lime zest, chili powder, salt, and pepper to create a dry rub.

2 Pat dry the salmon filets and season with the dry rub.

3 Heat the oil in a large skillet and place the salmon in the pan. Cook for 4 to 5 minutes on each side or until the salmon is tender and flakes easily.

4 In another bowl, add cubed avocado, onion, cilantro, lime juice, and salt and pepper to taste. Mix to combine.

5 Serve the rice in shallow bowls. Place salmon on top of the rice and top with the avocado salsa.

6 Garnish with more cilantro or lime juice, if desired.

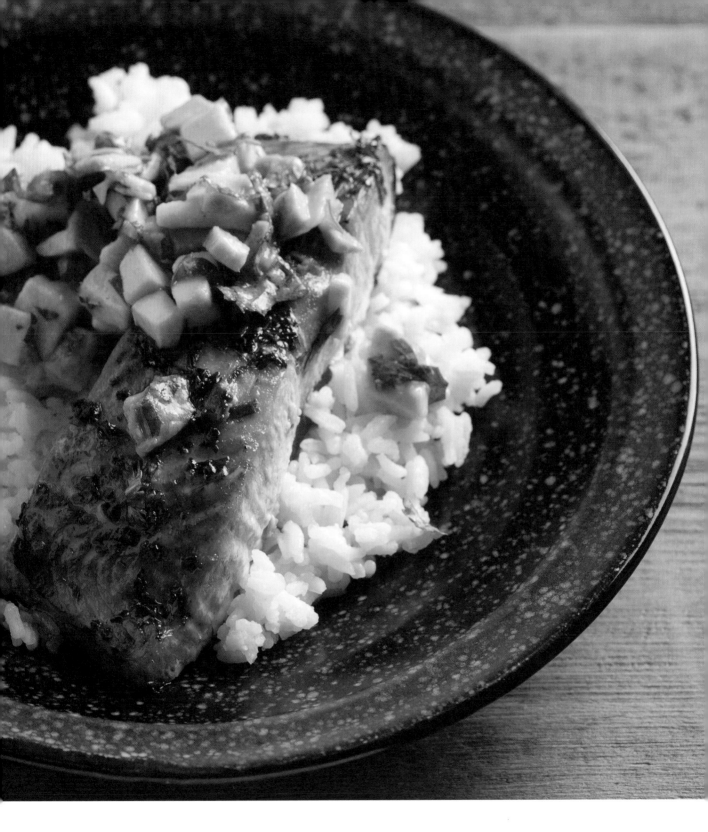

Avocado Salsa

2 Hass avocados, cubed

¼ cup diced red onion

¼ cup chopped cilantro

Juice of 2 limes

Salt and pepper, to taste

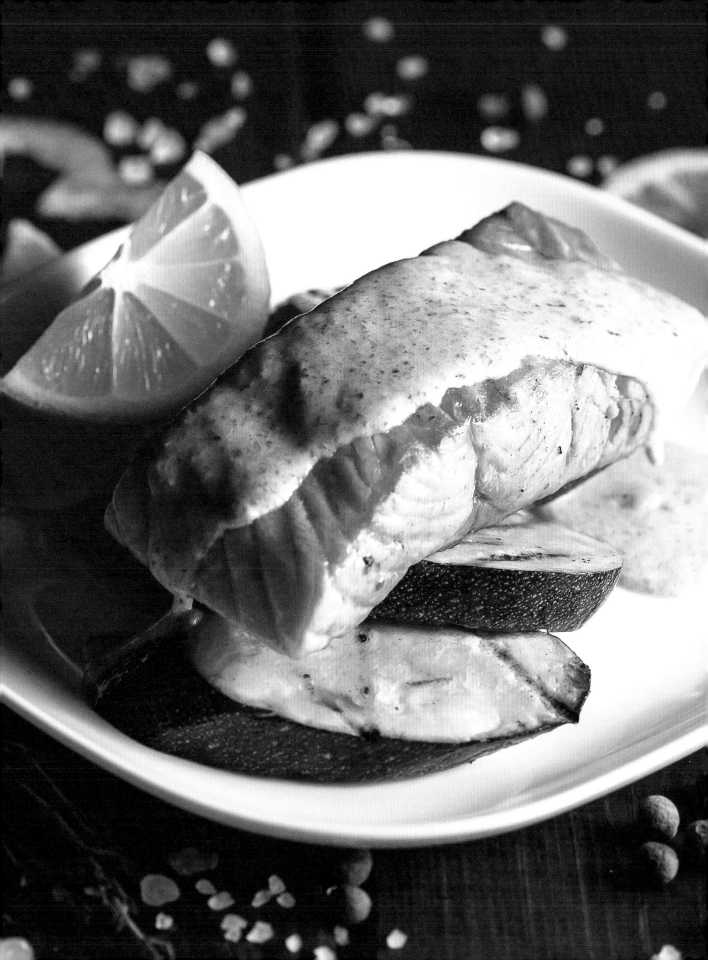

Savory Baked Salmon & Zucchini

This recipe is great for busy nights. Throw everything together in a pan, place it in the oven, and you have a quick and easy meal that serves you plenty of anti-inflammatory micro and macronutrients.

INGREDIENTS

2-3 medium zucchinis, chopped in half moons or quartered

4 (3 oz.) fillets wild-caught salmon

3-4 tablespoons extra-virgin olive oil

1 teaspoon sea salt

4 garlic cloves, minced

1 teaspoon lemon zest

½ teaspoon dried chives

½ teaspoon dried parsley

½ teaspoon black pepper

Juice of ½ large lemon

INSTRUCTIONS

1 Preheat the oven to 400°F.

2 Place the salmon fillets in the middle of a large baking sheet and spread zucchini pieces around the salmon.

3 Drizzle olive oil over the salmon and zucchini.

4 Put the seasoning ingredients in a small bowl and mix to combine.

5 Season the salmon and zucchini with the seasoning and place the baking sheet in the oven for 15 minutes.

6 Remove the pan from the oven and sprinkle the salmon and zucchini with lemon juice. Serve.

Pan-Fried Teriyaki Salmon

This is a great alternative to a teriyaki meal from your local take-out restaurant. This simple teriyaki salmon is made from whole foods that support your health instead of inflammatory preservatives, sugars, or flavor enhancers.

INGREDIENTS

4 (3 oz.) fillets wild-caught salmon

½ cup coconut aminos, divided

1 tablespoon sesame oil

1 teaspoon garlic, minced

¼ cup scallions

½ teaspoon ground ginger

1 tablespoon rice vinegar

Sea salt, to taste

Pinch of crushed red pepper (optional)

2 tablespoons avocado oil

1 teaspoon arrowroot flour

INSTRUCTIONS

1 Place the salmon in a large resealable bag and add ¼ cup coconut aminos, sesame oil, garlic, scallions, ginger, rice vinegar, salt, and crushed red pepper, if using.

2 Place the salmon in the fridge overnight or for at least 1 hour before cooking.

3 Heat the avocado oil in a large skillet over high heat. Once the oil is hot, add the salmon and marinade into the pan. Cook the salmon for about 4 to 6 minutes on each side or until the salmon flakes off with a fork and the middle is no longer dark pink.

4 Remove the salmon from the pan. Add the remaining ¼ cup of aminos and the arrowroot flour to the pan. Whisk until the sauce begins to thicken.

5 Add salmon back to the skillet to coat and serve with your favorite vegetable, rice, or cauliflower rice.

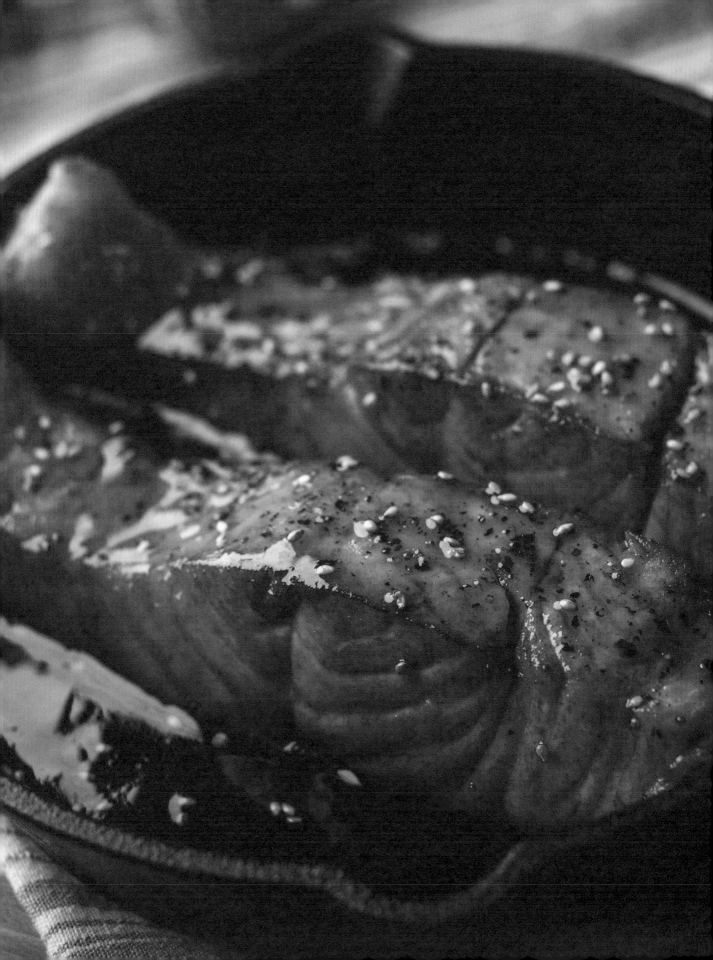

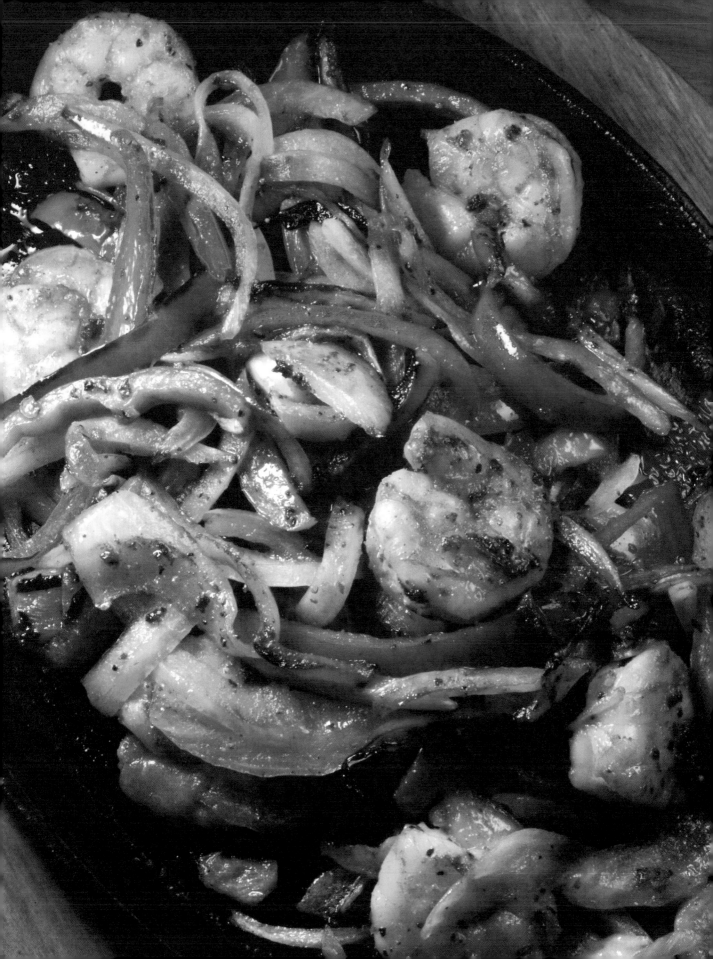

Shrimp Fajitas

This recipe for shrimp fajitas makes it easy to enjoy a flavorful meal and a functional immune system that keeps inflammation at bay. Shrimp is a great source of selenium, B12, and iron, while the onions and peppers provide tons of nutrients and phytonutrients.

INGREDIENTS

2 tablespoons avocado oil, divided

1 lb. shrimp, peeled and deveined

1 tablespoon grass-fed butter or ghee

2 tablespoons Taco Seasoning (see recipe on page 97)

Juice of ½ lime

1 medium red bell pepper, julienned

1 medium green bell pepper, julienned

1 medium orange bell pepper, julienned

1 medium yellow onion, sliced

1 Hass avocado, sliced

⅓ cup cilantro, chopped

INSTRUCTIONS

1   Heat the avocado oil in a large skillet. Once hot, add the shrimp, butter, and 1 tablespoon Taco Seasoning and sauté for 5 minutes or until the shrimp is pink and cooked. Drizzle with lime juice.

2   Remove the shrimp and heat the remaining avocado oil in the pan. Add peppers and onion along with 1 tablespoon Taco Seasoning. Sauté for about 10 minutes or until the vegetables are tender.

3   Remove the peppers from the heat and return the shrimp to the pan. Toss to combine

4   Serve the fajitas with non-GMO corn tortillas or grain-free tortillas (I like Siete tortillas). Top with avocado and cilantro.

Instant Pot Spanish Chicken Stew

This is the perfect recipe when you're short on time. You can also make this recipe in a slow cooker, just add all of the ingredients and let it cook for 8 hours.

INGREDIENTS

2 tablespoons avocado oil

2 lbs. boneless chicken breasts, cut into chunks

2 teaspoons ground cumin

1 teaspoon sea salt

1 teaspoon garlic powder

½ tablespoon dried oregano

1 teaspoon garlic, minced

1 medium yellow onion, sliced

4 medium red potatoes, cut into chunks

1 cup jarred roasted red pepper, sliced

2 medium carrots, cut into chunks

¼ cup sugar-free salsa verde

1½ cups chicken broth

1 cup tomato sauce

⅓ cup loosely packed fresh cilantro, finely chopped, for garnish

INSTRUCTIONS

1 Turn on the Sauté setting on your Instant Pot. Add the avocado oil.

2 Once heated, add the chicken, spices, and minced garlic and sauté for about 2 minutes.

3 Add the onions, potatoes, roasted red peppers, and carrots to the pot. Sauté for another 2 minutes.

4 Add the sugar-free salsa, chicken broth, and tomato sauce. Close the lid on your Instant Pot and switch to the Pressure Cook/Manual setting.

5 Cook the stew for 20 minutes and then natural release for 5 minutes. Then, press the Quick-Release button, garnish with the cilantro, and serve with a side salad or your preferred rice.

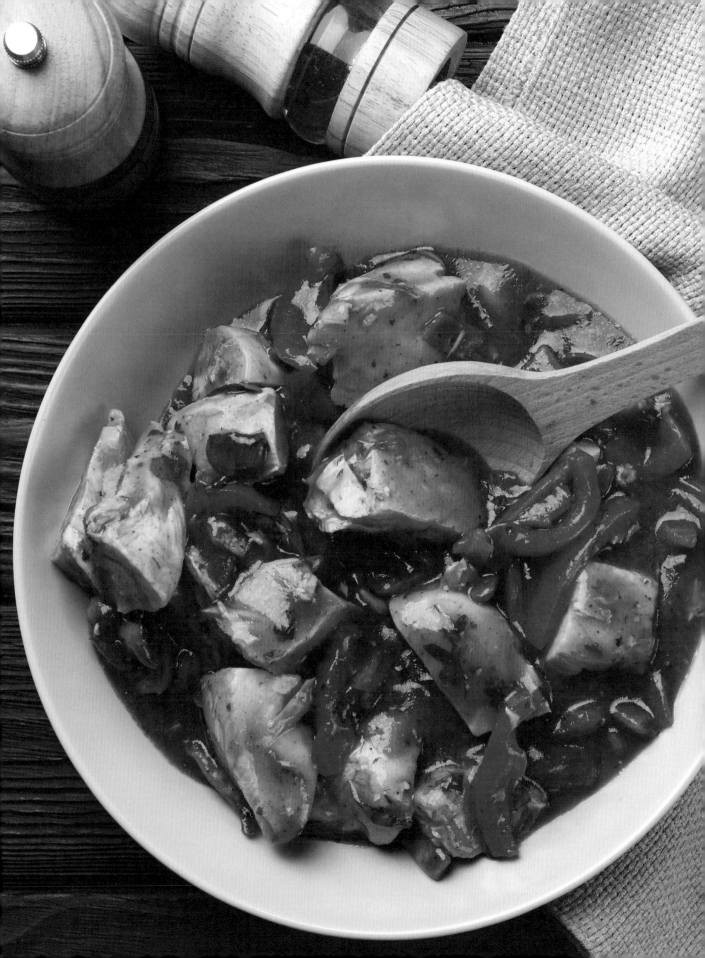

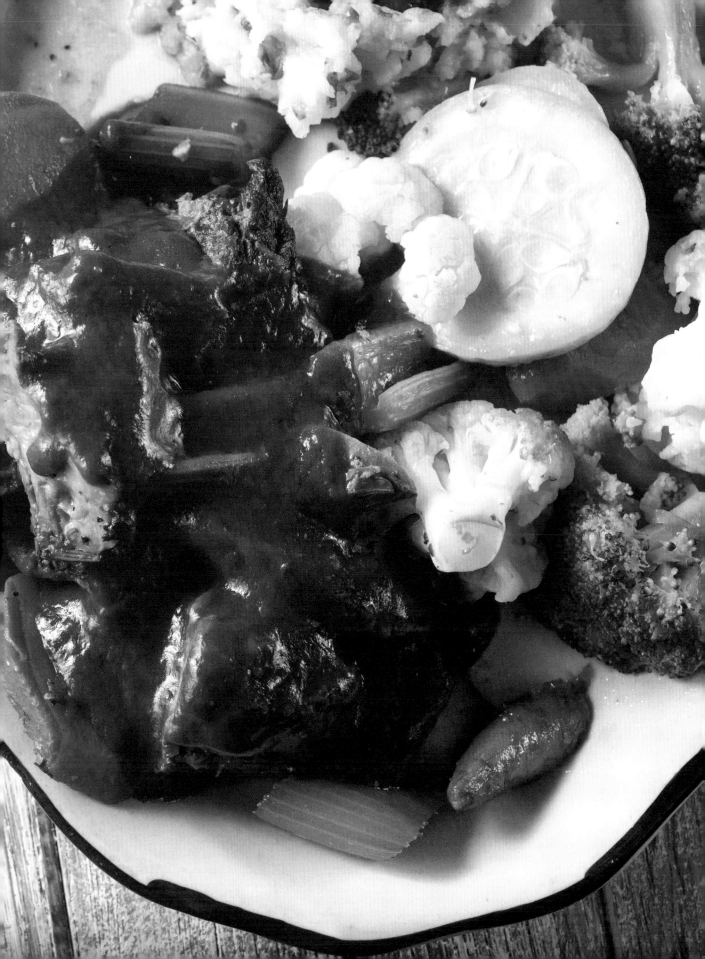

Slow Cooker Pot Roast with Roasted Veggies

Slow cooked meats are the best. Just set it, forget it, and come back 8 hours later to a whole meal. You can use this roast as a protein addition to any salad or veggie side dish. The recipe also calls for bone broth, which in an incredible source of numerous vitamins, minerals, and amino acids that support your immune system and digestive health.

INGREDIENTS

2 tablespoons onion powder

2 tablespoons garlic powder

2 teaspoons cumin

2 tablespoons sea salt

1 tablespoon Italian seasoning

1 tablespoon black pepper

4 lbs. beef chuck roast or shoulder roast

1 large yellow onion, sliced

1 cup beef bone broth

2 cups broccoli florets

2 cups cauliflower florets

2 tablespoons olive oil

INSTRUCTIONS

1 In a small bowl, add the spices and mix to combine.

2 Place the roast in the slow cooker with sliced onion. Use about half of the dry seasoning mixture and season the roast well. Pour the broth over roast. Close the lid and cook on low for 8 hours.

3 When the roast is almost done, preheat the oven to 400°F.

4 Place the vegetables on a baking sheet with the remainder of the dry seasoning and drizzle with olive oil. Combine the seasoning and vegetables and mix well.

5 Put the baking sheet in the oven for about 20 to 25 minutes.

6 Transfer the beef from the slow cooker to a cutting board and shred the meat with 2 forks. Place meat back in slow cooker.

7 Serve the roast with roasted vegetables.

Marinated Flank Steak with Asparagus

Marinating tough cuts of meat like flank steak in an acidic marinade helps break down the proteins for a tender and juicy steak. This recipe is a hearty meal that doesn't compromise your nutritional goals.

INGREDIENTS

⅓ cup coconut aminos

1 tablespoon spicy brown mustard

1 tablespoon raw apple cider vinegar

4 garlic cloves, minced

½ teaspoon onion powder

½ teaspoon garlic powder

¼ teaspoon smoked paprika

½ teaspoon salt, plus more to taste

½ teaspoon black pepper, plus more to taste

1 tablespoon chopped chives

1½ lbs. grass-fed flank steak

2-3 tablespoons grass-fed butter

1 bunch asparagus, fibrous ends removed

1 tablespoon olive oil

¼ teaspoon lemon zest

INSTRUCTIONS

1 In a large resealable bag or Tupperware container, combine the aminos, mustard, apple cider vinegar, garlic, spices, chives, and flank steak. Let the steak marinate for at least 3 to 4 hours or overnight before grilling.

2 Heat the butter in a large cast-iron skillet. Once the butter is melted, add the steak and cook for about 4 to 5 minutes on each side.

3 In a separate skillet, heat the olive oil. Once the skillet is hot, add the asparagus and salt and pepper to taste. Sauté for about 8 to 10 minutes.

4 Garnish the steak with lemon zest and serve with asparagus.

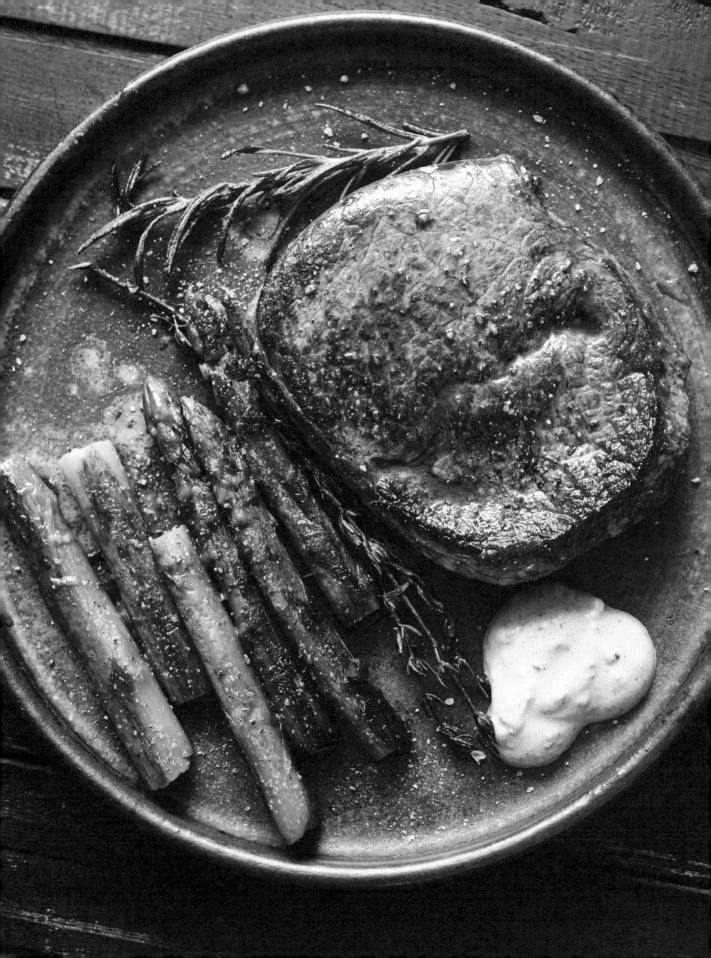

Veggie Meatloaf

Let's be clear, this is not a vegetarian meatloaf—but it does include various vegetables that hold the antioxidants, phytonutrients, and essential minerals you need to support your immune system. Sourcing grass-fed meat amps up the nutritional value of this meatloaf by adding additional omega-3 fatty acids.

INGREDIENTS

1 tablespoon olive oil

⅓ cup diced yellow onion

⅓ cup diced mushrooms

⅓ cup diced celery

1 cup chopped spinach

½ cup tomato sauce

2 tablespoons tomato paste, divided

1 teaspoon apple cider vinegar

1 tablespoon coconut aminos

Salt, to taste, plus ½ teaspoon

Black pepper, to taste, plus ¼ teaspoon

¼ cup chopped fresh parsley

2 lbs. ground beef

2 whole pasture-raised eggs, beaten

½ cup almond flour

INSTRUCTIONS

1 Preheat the oven to 350°F.

2 In a small skillet, heat the oil and add the onion, mushrooms, celery, and spinach. Sauté for about 3 to 5 minutes. Remove the mixture from the pan and let it cool.

3 In a small bowl, combine the tomato sauce, 1 tablespoon tomato paste, apple cider vinegar, coconut aminos, and salt and pepper to taste. Set the bowl aside.

4 In a large mixing bowl, combine the vegetables, fresh parsley, ½ teaspoon salt, ¼ teaspoon pepper, 1 tablespoon tomato paste, beef, eggs, and almond flour. Using clean hands or a spoon, mix until well combined.

5 Place the meat mixture on a sheet pan and shape the mixture into a rectangular loaf.

6 Bake the meatloaf for about an hour or until the internal temperature reaches 160°F.

7 Let the meatloaf cool for about 10 to 15 minutes before slicing.

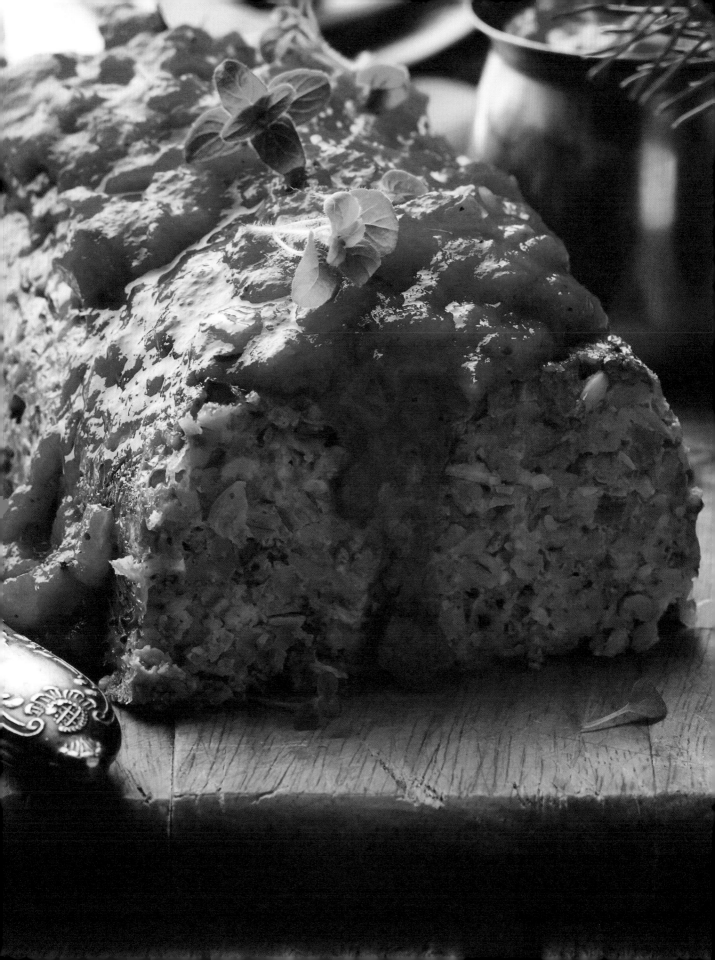

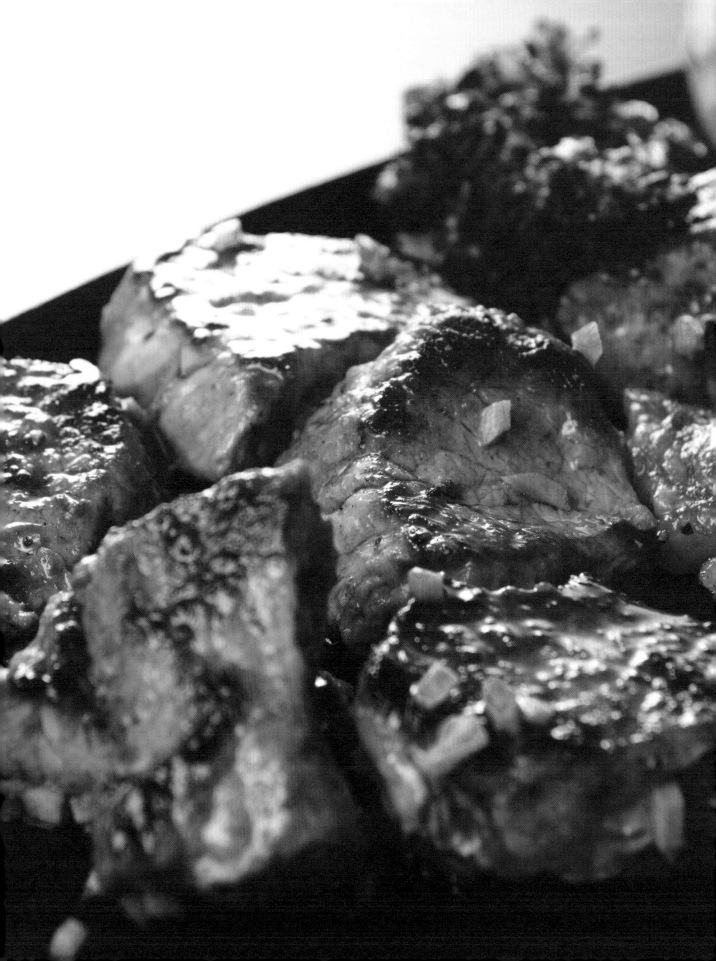

Savory Herb Steak Chunks

You don't need tons of time or skill to cook a satisfying and nutritious steak dinner. Steak is a savory protein that will go perfectly with your favorite vegetable or atop a salad.

INGREDIENTS

½ teaspoon salt

½ teaspoon black pepper

3 tablespoons unsalted butter

6 cloves garlic, minced

2 tablespoons chopped fresh parsley

2 tablespoons chopped fresh chives

½ tablespoon avocado oil

1½ lbs. grass-fed sirloin or ribeye steak, cut into 1-inch chunks

INSTRUCTIONS

1 In a small food processor, combine the salt, pepper, butter, garlic, parsley, and chives. Process the mixture until well combined.

2 Heat the avocado oil in a medium skillet on high heat. Add the steak and sauté for about 4 to 5 minutes.

3 Remove the steak from the pan and add the butter mixture. Once melted and aromatic, return the steak to the pan and toss well to coat.

Meatballs with Spaghetti Squash

This is almost a one-pan meal! Spaghetti squash is an excellent source of fiber, vitamin C, and beta-carotene, all of which strengthen your immune system's response to inflammatory triggers. Grass-fed beef also adds additional anti-inflammatory omega-3 fatty acids.

INGREDIENTS

1½ lbs. grass-fed beef

¼ cup almond flour

1 teaspoon garlic powder

½ teaspoon dried parsley

½ teaspoon dried oregano

1 teaspoon onion powder

1 teaspoon sea salt

½ teaspoon black pepper

1 tablespoon grated Parmesan cheese (omit if sensitive to dairy)

1-2 whole pasture-raised eggs, beaten

1 spaghetti squash

1 tablespoon olive oil

1 (24 oz.) jar sugar-free pasta sauce

INSTRUCTIONS

1   Preheat oven to 400°F.

2   In a mixing bowl, combine the beef, flour, garlic powder, parsley, oregano, onion powder, salt, pepper, Parmesan cheese, and egg(s).

3   Use clean hands to combine the ingredients and form meatballs about the size of a golf ball.

4   Place each meatball on a greased baking sheet and cook the meatballs in the oven for about 10 minutes.

5   Slice the spaghetti squash in half lengthwise and scoop out the seeds and ribbing. For ease, poke holes in the squash and microwave for 5 to 7 minutes.

Continued...

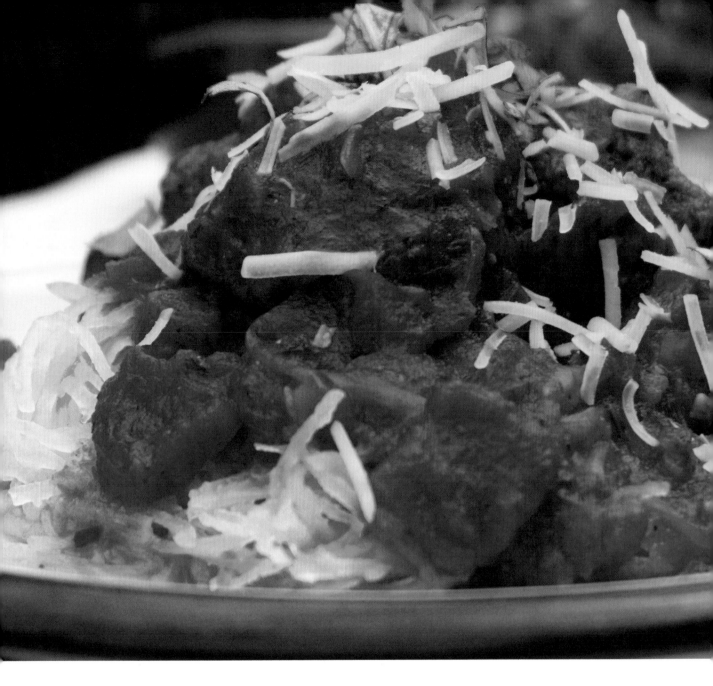

6　Drizzle the inside of the squash with olive oil and sprinkle with salt and pepper. Place the spaghetti squash cut side down on the baking sheet. Roast for 30 to 45 minutes or until lightly browned on the outside and the inside is easy to pierce with a fork. Remove the pan from the oven and let cool.

7　After the meatballs have cooked for 10 minutes, remove the pan from the oven and pour the sauce over the meatballs. Place the pan back into the oven for another 5 to 7 minutes.

8　Once the squash has cooled, use a fork to scrape out the flesh and shred bigger pieces. It should easily come apart and look like spaghetti.

9　Spoon the meatballs over the spaghetti squash.

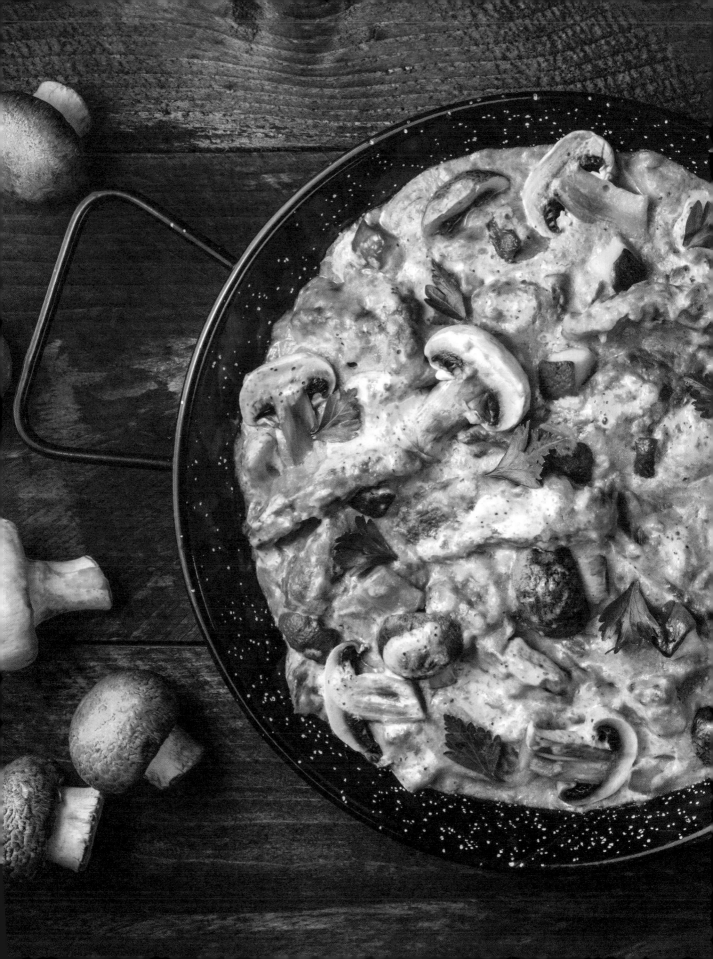

Slow Cooker Beef Stroganoff

This is another great slow cooker recipe that provides all of the quality protein and fat you need to stay full, satisfied, and properly nourished.

INGREDIENTS

1½ lbs. grass-fed sirloin steak tips or stew steak

1 medium yellow onion, sliced

5 garlic cloves, minced

2 cups sliced mushrooms

1½ cup beef broth

¼ cup coconut aminos

¼ cup red wine vinegar

1 teaspoon onion powder

1 teaspoon garlic powder

½ teaspoon sea salt

¼ teaspoon black pepper

½ cup canned coconut milk

⅓ cup chopped fresh parsley, for garnish

INSTRUCTIONS

1 Place the steak, onions, garlic, and mushrooms in the slow cooker.

2 In a shallow bowl, mix the broth, coconut aminos, red wine vinegar, onion powder, garlic powder, salt, and pepper.

3 Pour the mixture on top of the beef and vegetables. Close the lid and set to cook on low for 6 hours. After 6 hours, open the lid and stir the beef. Add coconut milk and stir.

4 Close lid and let the beef cook for another 50 minutes.

5 Serve with gluten-free noodles or over rice and garnish with parsley.

Slow Cooker Beef Stew

If you haven't figured it out by now, I'm a huge fan of slow cooked beef. Slow cooked meals are delicious and nutritious. This recipe also calls for bone broth, which is like gold for your immune system, while the vegetables add supportive vitamins and minerals.

INGREDIENTS

2 tablespoons olive oil

1½ lbs. boneless beef chuck, cubed

3 cups beef bone broth

4 large carrots, chopped

1 medium onion, chopped

2-3 cups baby melody potatoes

1 teaspoon garlic, minced

1 lb. cremini mushrooms, chopped

2 tablespoons coconut aminos (or compliant Worcestershire sauce)

2 tablespoons tomato paste

1 teaspoon dried oregano

3 teaspoons Italian seasoning

2 teaspoons paprika

1 teaspoon sea salt

½ teaspoon black pepper

1 bay leaf

INSTRUCTIONS

1   Heat the olive oil in a cast-iron skillet on high heat. Sear the meat for about 30 seconds on each side.

2   Add the beef and the remaining ingredients into the slow cooker. Stir everything together and cook the stew on low for 8 hours.

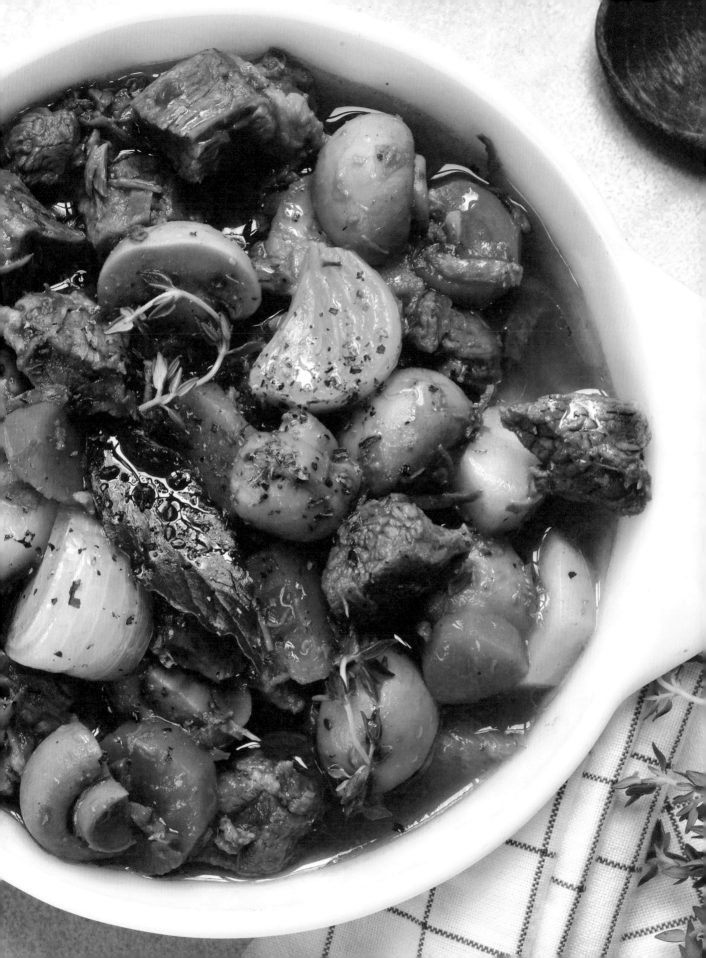

Asian Lettuce Tacos

This fresh and flavorful meal has all of the quality protein,
fat, and fiber you need to stay satisfied and nourished.

INGREDIENTS

½ tablespoon sesame seed oil

1 tablespoon avocado oil

2 garlic cloves, minced

1 lb. grass-fed ground beef

1 red bell pepper, diced

1 small yellow onion, diced

¼ cup coconut aminos

1 tablespoon rice vinegar or
apple cider vinegar

¼ teaspoon ground ginger

¼ teaspoon crushed red pepper
(optional)

¼ cup roasted cashews, chopped

6 romaine lettuce leaves or
butter leaf lettuce

¼ cup scallions, chopped,
for garnish

INSTRUCTIONS

1 In a large skillet, heat the sesame seed oil and avocado oil over medium-high heat and add the minced garlic along with the ground beef.

2 Sauté the beef and continue to break down the larger pieces. Cook for about 8 minutes or until browned.

3 Remove the beef and add the red bell pepper and onion. Cook for about 3 minutes, then add the aminos, vinegar, ginger, and crushed red pepper. Cook for another 2 to 3 minutes and add the cashews.

4 Remove the beef mix from the heat and serve over lettuce leaves with scallions.

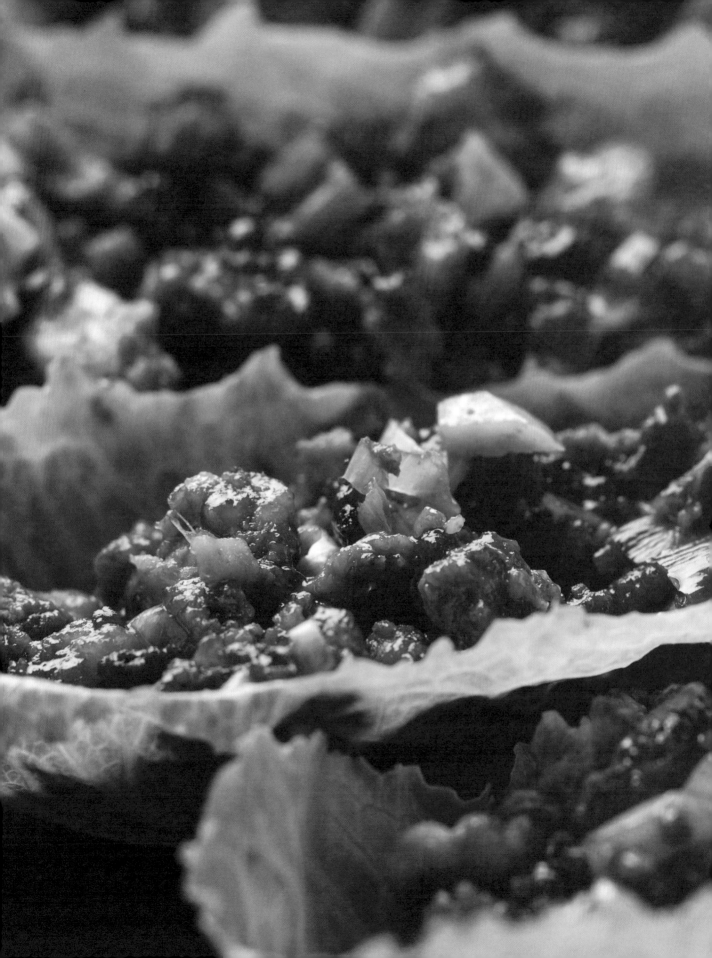

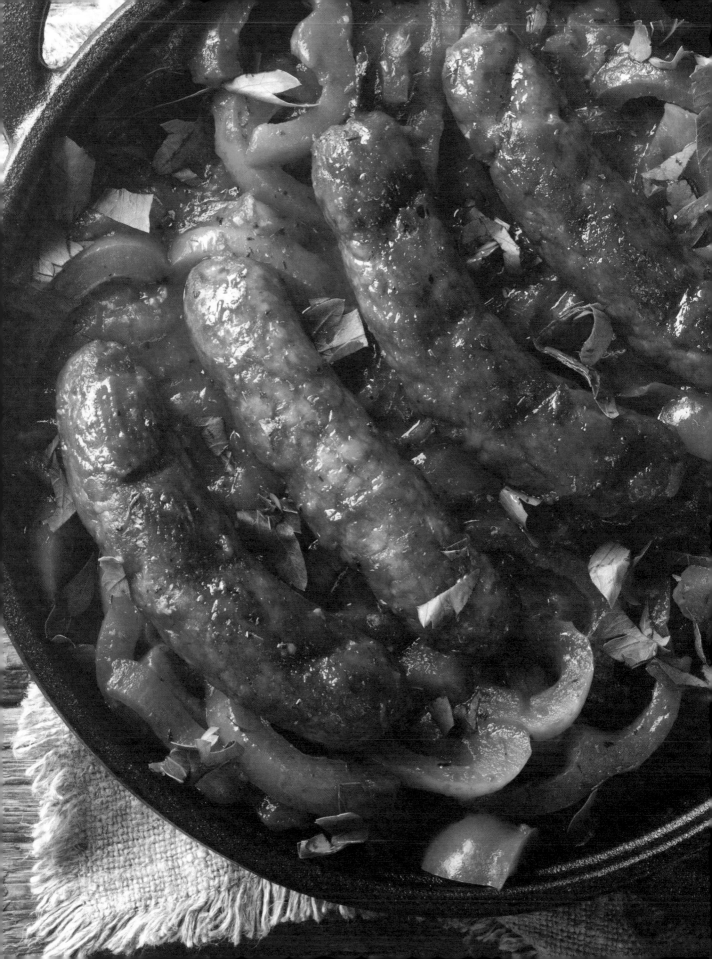

Italian Sausage & Peppers

This is a go-to one-pan meal. Pork has plenty of essential nutrients that support your immune system, including B vitamins, zinc, and potassium.

INGREDIENTS

2 teaspoons olive oil

1 lb. sweet Italian sausage links or ground sweet Italian sausage

3 garlic cloves, minced

1 medium yellow onion, sliced

1 medium red bell pepper, sliced

1 medium green bell pepper, sliced

1 medium yellow bell pepper, sliced

¼ teaspoon garlic powder

Salt and pepper, to taste

¼ cup chopped fresh parsley or chives, for garnish (optional)

INSTRUCTIONS

1 In a large cast-iron skillet, heat the olive oil. Once hot, add sausage and sauté for about 10 to 12 minutes or until brown and crispy. Remove sausage from pan

2 In the same skillet, add the garlic along with all of the peppers and onion. Stir in the garlic powder.

3 Cook the peppers and onion until tender. Add salt and pepper to taste.

4 Once the vegetables are cooked, return the sausage to the pan and toss to combine. Remove from heat.

5 Garnish with fresh parsley or chives and serve over your favorite vegetables, gluten-free bread, or wrap.

Slow Cooker Pork Roast

Pork shoulder and pork butt are great cuts in general, but in a slow cooker the end result is the most tender meat you can imagine. Using bone-in cuts also adds extra nutrients like glutamine, glycine, magnesium, calcium, and other essential amino acids and minerals that support your immune system against inflammation.

INGREDIENTS

3–4 lbs. skinless, bone-in pork butt or pork shoulder

1 teaspoon cumin

1 teaspoon garlic powder

1 teaspoon onion powder

1 teaspoon salt, divided

1 teaspoon dried oregano

1 medium yellow onion, sliced

5 garlic cloves, minced

¼ cup fresh-squeezed orange juice

1 cup bone broth

2 limes, sliced

Fresh lime juice, for garnish

¼ cup chopped fresh cilantro, for garnish

INSTRUCTIONS

1 Pat the pork dry with paper towels.

2 In a small bowl, mix the cumin, garlic powder, onion powder, ½ teaspoon salt, and dried oregano and stir to combine. Rub seasoning on the pork, covering all sides.

3 Place the pork in the slow cooker along with the onion, garlic cloves, orange juice, ½ teaspoon salt, and bone broth. Cook on low for 8 to 10 hours.

4 Once the pork is finished, remove it from the slow cooker and place it onto a cutting board. Use 2 forks to shred pork.

5 Serve over white rice, brown rice, cauliflower rice, or corn tortilla. Garnish with fresh lime juice and cilantro.

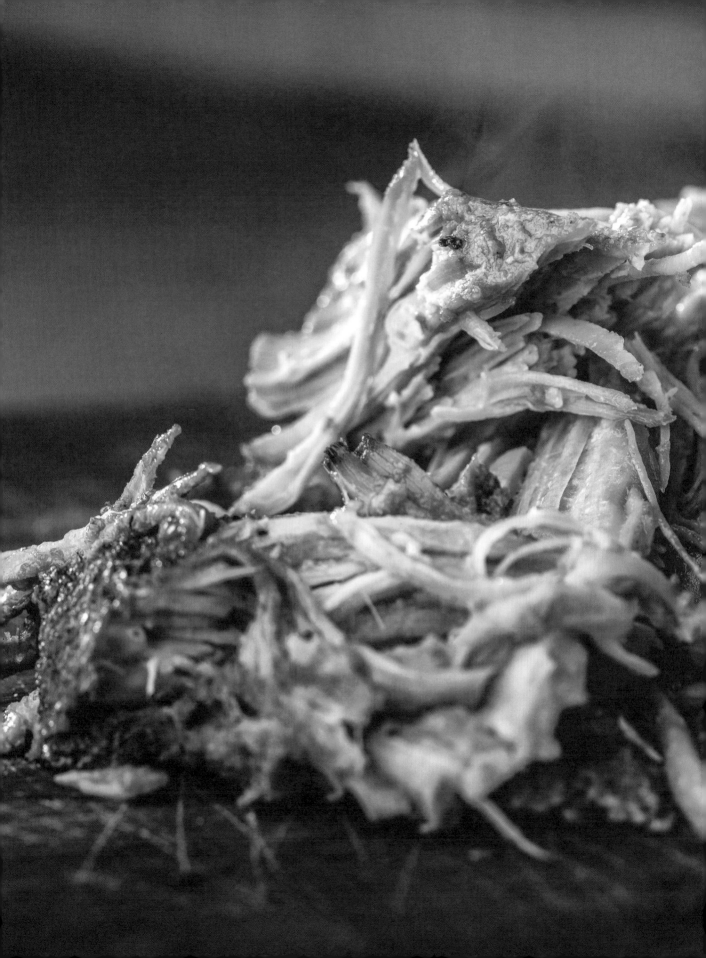

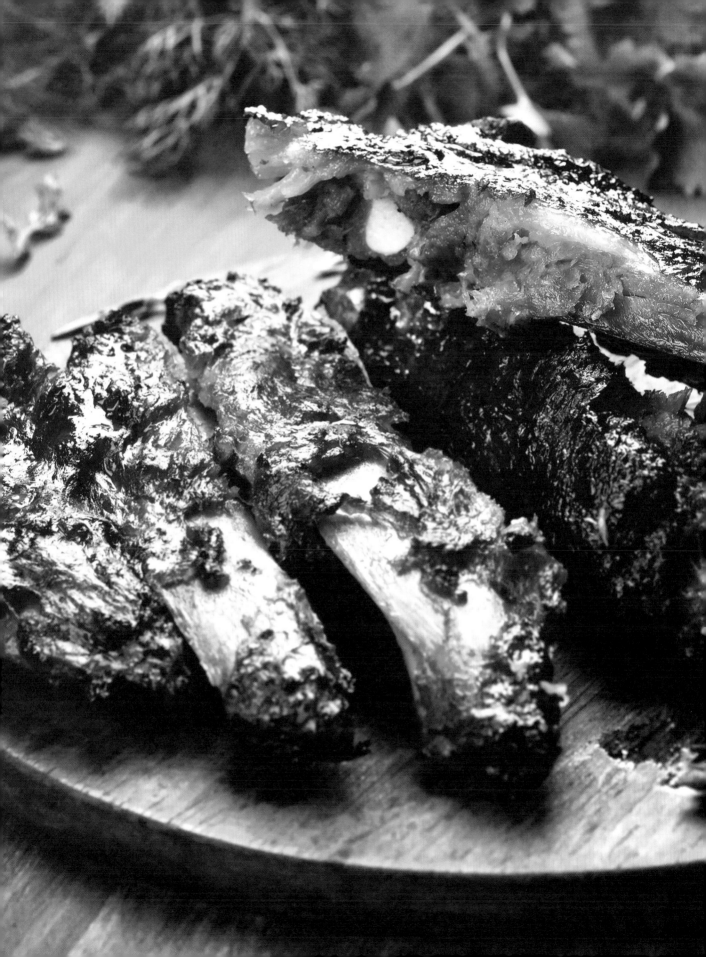

BBQ Ribs

Most people believe that ribs are off the food list when it comes to eating nutritious foods. Luckily, not only do ribs provide zinc, iron, and B vitamins, this recipe also calls for a BBQ sauce that isn't loaded with inflammatory sugars.

INGREDIENTS

1 rack pork ribs

2 teaspoons salt

2 teaspoons black pepper

2 teaspoons smoked paprika

1 teaspoon garlic powder

1 teaspoon onion powder

½ cup Homemade BBQ Sauce (see recipe on page 101)

INSTRUCTIONS

1 Preheat the oven to 275°F.

2 Remove the membrane from the back of the ribs, if not removed already. Rinse the ribs in cold water and pat dry.

3 In a small bowl, combine the salt, pepper, smoked paprika, garlic powder, and onion powder. Season both sides of the ribs with the dry seasoning.

4 Place the ribs on a rimmed baking sheet. Cover the baking sheet tightly with aluminum foil and bake for 3 to 4 hours. The meat should easily come off the bone.

5 Remove ribs from the oven and set oven to high broil. Brush ribs with BBQ sauce and place ribs back in the oven for 2-3 minutes. Watch carefully to avoid burning. Remove from oven and serve.

Sweet & Savory Pork Chops

I always like to have something sweet with pork chops. This recipe is a great combination of sweet and savory. Plus, the sweetness from the apples reduces cravings for inflammatory sweets after dinner.

INGREDIENTS

¼ teaspoon salt

Pinch or ⅛ teaspoon black pepper

1 teaspoon onion powder

½ teaspoon cinnamon

4 bone-in pork chops

2 medium honey crisp or gala apples, sliced

1 teaspoon fresh lemon juice

3 tablespoons ghee or grass-fed butter

1 small red onion, sliced thin

1 teaspoon spicy brown mustard

1½ tablespoons Italian seasoning

INSTRUCTIONS

1 Preheat the oven to 375°F.

2 In a small bowl, mix the salt, pepper, onion powder, and cinnamon. Season both sides of each pork chop with the spice mixture.

3 In a larger bowl, combine the sliced apples with lemon juice.

4 In a large cast-iron skillet, heat half of the ghee or butter. Once melted, add the pork chops and brown on both sides for about 3 to 5 minutes.

5 Remove the pork chops from the pan and melt the remaining ghee or butter. Add the apples and onion and season with a pinch of salt, a pinch of pepper, the spicy brown mustard, and Italian seasoning. Sauté for 5 minutes.

6 Add the pork back to the cast-iron skillet and carefully place the skillet in the oven. Bake for 5 to 7 minutes or until an internal temperature of 145°F is reached.

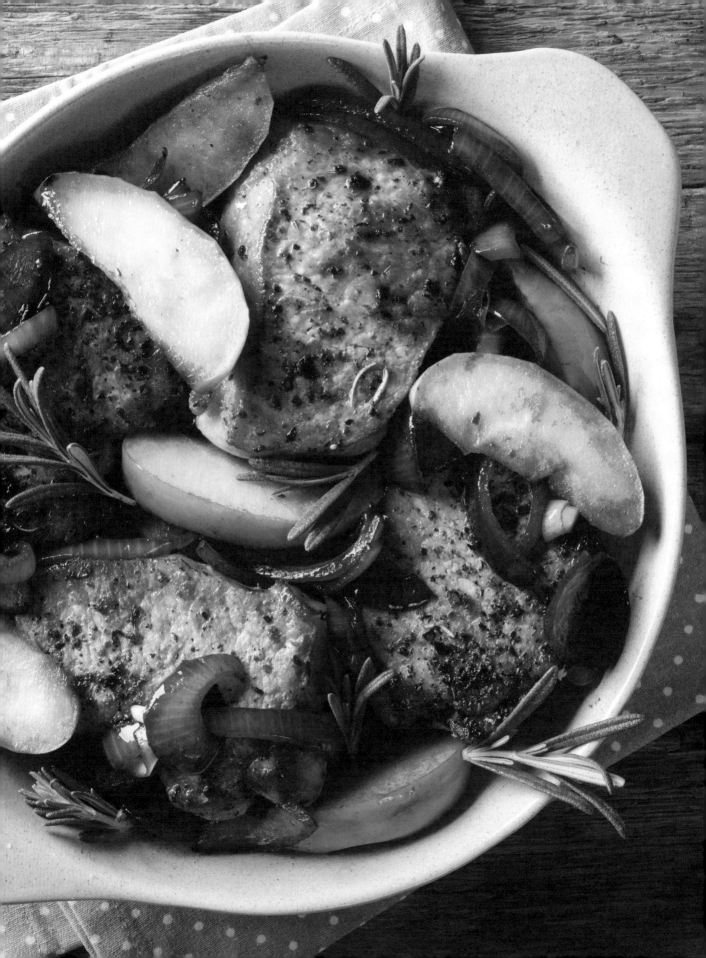

Apple Bacon Pork Tenderloin

This is a recipe seem fancy, but it is very simple to make. Serve this hearty meal with herbed potatoes and your favorite greens.

INGREDIENTS

1 lb. pork tenderloin

Salt and pepper, to taste

2 teaspoons Italian seasoning, divided

1 medium apple, roughly chopped

2 garlic cloves, minced

1 tablespoon Dijon mustard

1 tablespoon balsamic vinegar

8-10 strips humanely raised bacon, thinly cut

INSTRUCTIONS

1 Preheat the oven to 425°F.

2 Pat the pork dry with paper towels and season with salt and pepper and 1 teaspoon Italian seasoning.

3 In a food processor or blender, combine the apple, garlic, mustard, and balsamic vinegar. Process the mix until it is the consistency of a chunky apple sauce.

4 Lay the bacon slices on a baking sheet, slightly overlapping one another. Place the tenderloin on top.

5 Spread apple mixture over tenderloin and then wrap bacon over the tenderloin.

6 Roast for 20 minutes or until it reaches an internal temperature of 145°F.

Optional: If you'd like crispier bacon, turn on the broiler for 1 to 2 minutes.

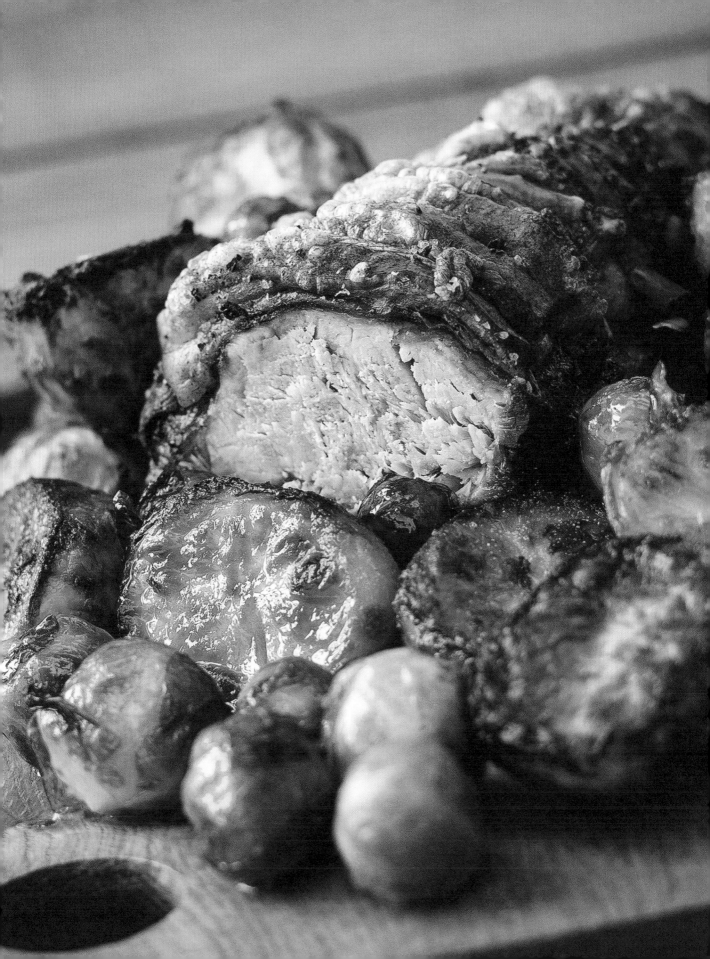

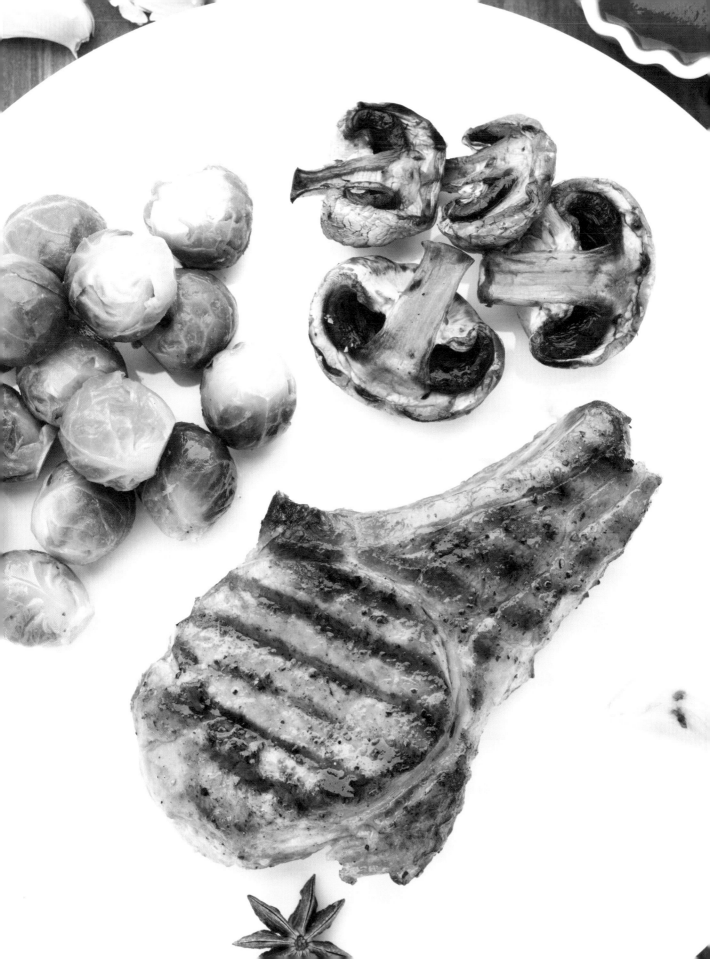

Sheet Pan Pork Dinner

This is a simple one-pan pork dinner that utilizes sulfur vegetables which support your body's natural detox system and reduce inflammation related to toxin overload.

INGREDIENTS

4 bone-in pork chops

Juice of 1 lemon

1 teaspoon garlic, minced

1 teaspoon Italian seasoning

1 tablespoon chopped fresh parsley

Cooking spray

2 cups halved Brussels sprouts

2 cups cubed pears, cubed

2 tablespoons olive oil

Salt and pepper, to taste

Pinch of cinnamon

INSTRUCTIONS

1 Preheat the oven to 425°F.

2 Pat the pork dry with a paper towel. In a separate bowl, mix the lemon juice, garlic, Italian seasoning, and parsley. Coat the pork chops in seasoning.

3 Lightly spray a large rimmed baking sheet with cooking spray. Place the pork chops on the baking sheet.

4 In a separate mixing bowl, combine the Brussels sprouts, pears, olive oil, salt, pepper, and cinnamon. Mix well.

5 Arrange the Brussels sprouts and pears around the pork chops on a baking sheet.

6 Place the baking sheet in the oven for about 20 minutes or until it reaches an internal temperature of 145°F.

Instant Pot Creamy Chicken & Rice

This is an incredibly satisfying and filling meal that takes little effort to make. The easier your meals can be, the more likely you are to stay on track to better health.

INGREDIENTS

2 large boneless skinless chicken breasts

¼ teaspoon salt

¼ teaspoon black pepper

¼ teaspoon onion powder

6 cups chicken stock or bone broth

1 cup wild rice, uncooked

½ tablespoon minced garlic

1 medium yellow onion, diced

3 large carrots, chopped

2 celery stalks, diced

2 teaspoons Italian seasoning

Continued...

INSTRUCTIONS

1 Add the chicken to the Instant Pot and season with salt, pepper, and onion powder.

2 Add the broth, rice, garlic, onion, carrots, celery, Italian seasoning, bay leaf, mushrooms, and broccoli florets.

3 Close the lid and set the Instant Pot to Pressure Cook/ Manual on High for 30 minutes.

4 In a small saucepan, combine the butter and coconut milk. Whisk until well combined.

5 Let your Instant Pot natural release for 5 minutes, then press the Quick-Release button. Add the coconut milk to the soup.

6 Garnish with black pepper and fresh parsley and serve soup in shallow bowls.

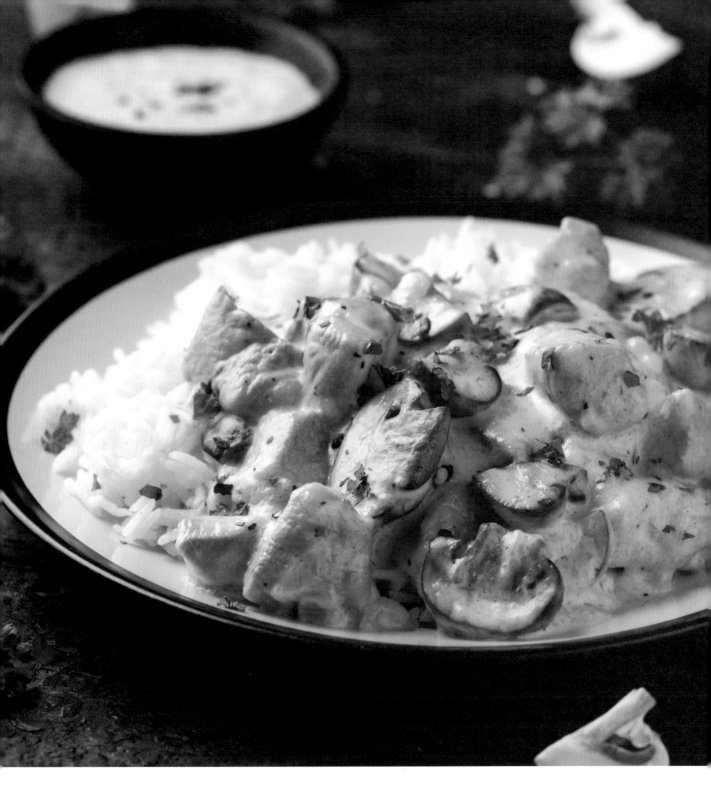

1 bay leaf

1 cup thinly sliced cremini mushrooms

1 cup broccoli florets

1 tablespoon grass-fed butter or ghee

1 (15 oz.) can full-fat coconut milk

¼ cup chopped fresh parsley, for garnish

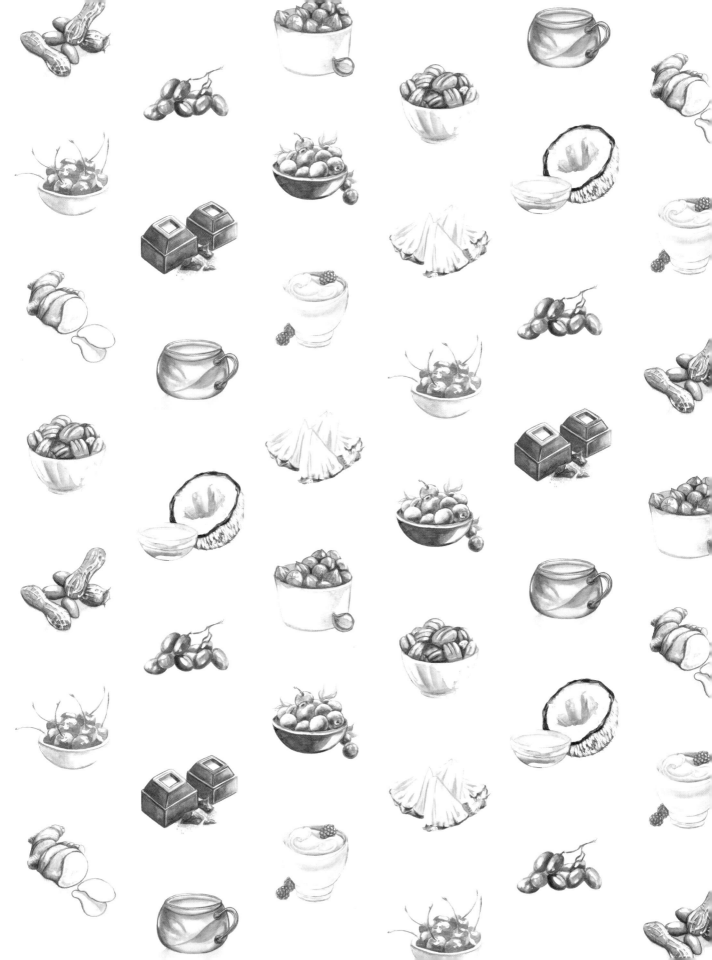

SWEETS

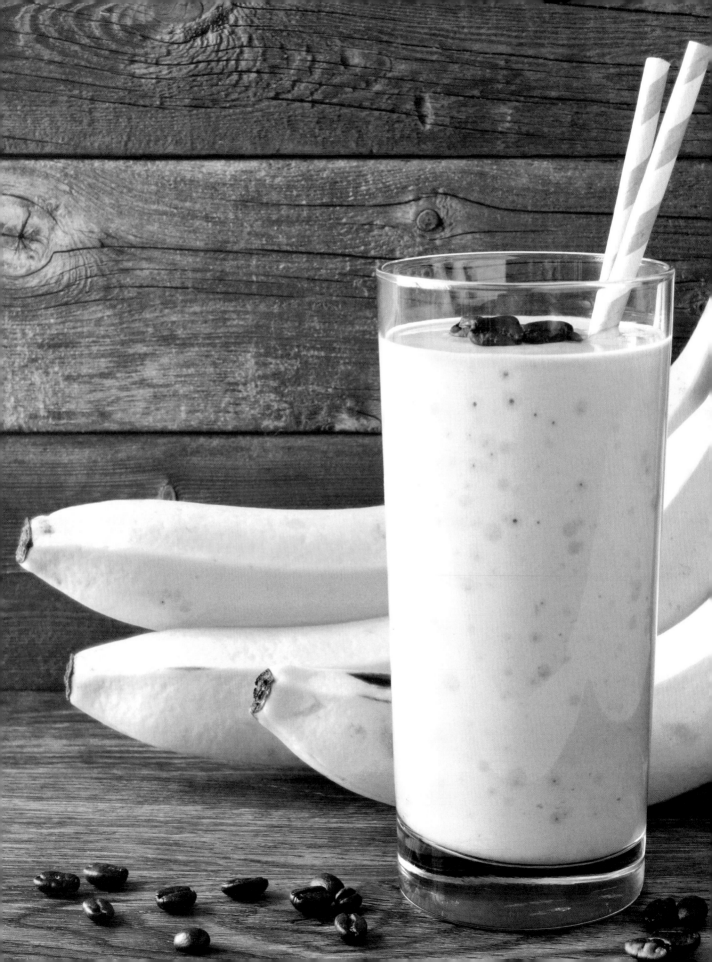

Wake Up Call Smoothie

This smoothie uses coffee to wake you up in the morning. The glycemic ingredients also balance each other out so you won't feel fatigued and hungry shortly after drinking it.

INGREDIENTS

1 cup strong coffee, cooled

1 frozen banana

2 tablespoons nut butter of choice

⅓ cup coconut milk

1 cup ice (optional)

INSTRUCTIONS

1 Add all of the ingredients into the blender and blend until the desired consistency is reached. Add ice for a thicker smoothie, if needed.

Berry Smoothie

Smoothies are nutrient-dense and provide you with plenty of antioxidants and phytonutrients that keep your immune system strong. To offset the increased sugar and carbohydrate content and avoid health issues associated with high blood sugar, it's important to add fat and protein to your smoothies.

INGREDIENTS

1 cup frozen mixed berries

2 tablespoons almond butter

1 scoop grass-fed collagen peptides

1 tablespoon chia seeds

1 frozen zucchini

1 cup almond milk

1 teaspoon ground flaxseed

INSTRUCTIONS

1 Add all of the ingredients into the blender and blend until the desired consistency is reached. For a thinner smoothie, add more almond milk or water.

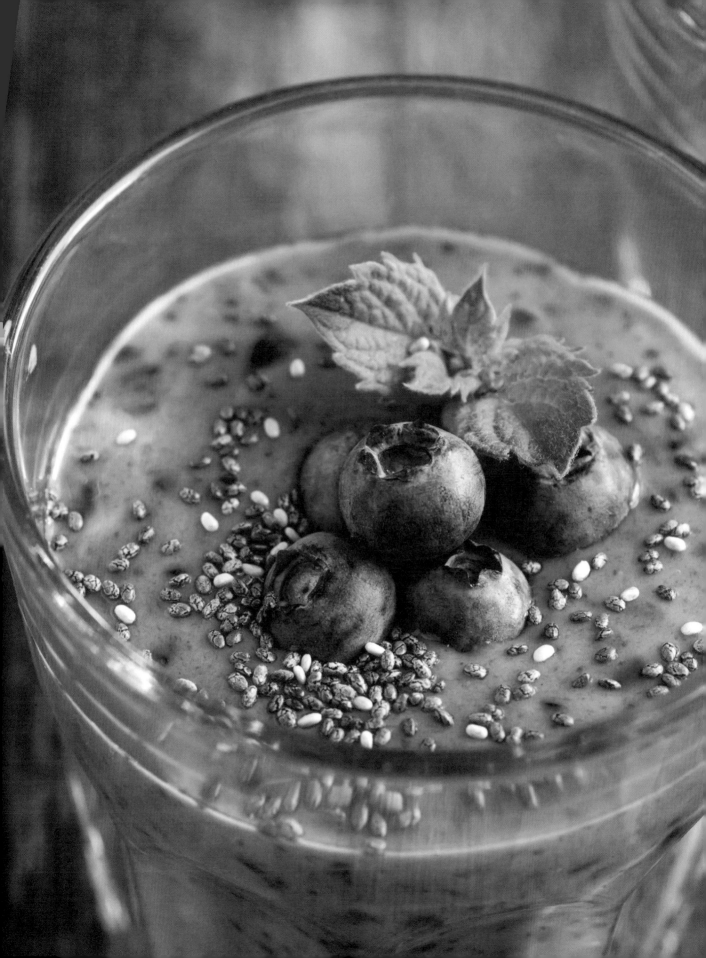

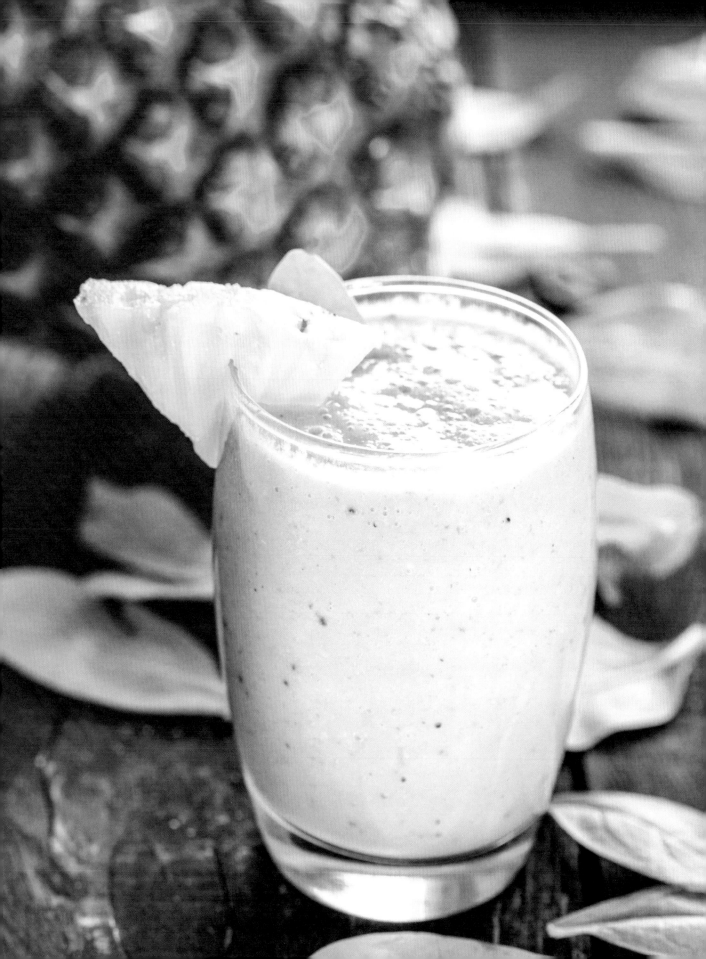

Green Smoothie

This smoothie is packed with tons of anti-inflammatory nutrients like folate, magnesium, B vitamins, glycine, potassium, and many others. We need all of these nutrients to work together to support our immune systems and prevent inflammatory triggers.

INGREDIENTS

1 cup almond milk or non-dairy milk of choice

2 cups kale

2 cups baby spinach

1 frozen banana or 1 cup frozen pineapple

1 scoop grass-fed collagen peptides

1 tablespoon chia seeds

1 tablespoon hemp seeds

INSTRUCTIONS

1 Add all of the ingredients into the blender and blend until the desired consistency is reached. If a thinner smoothie is desired, add more milk of choice or water.

Homemade Strawberry Jam

Most homemade jams contain a ton of sugar which triggers inflammatory pathways and promotes obesity, diabetes, autoimmunity, and other diseases. This recipe allows you to enjoy a delicious jam while also maintaining your health goals.

INGREDIENTS

3 cups fresh or frozen strawberries

2 tablespoons Lakanto Golden Monkfruit sweetener

1 tablespoon freshly-squeezed lemon juice

2 tablespoons chia seeds

INSTRUCTIONS

1 Place the fruit, sweetener, and lemon juice in a medium saucepan over medium-high heat and stir occasionally. Bring the mixture to a boil and then reduce the heat to a simmer.

2 Let the mixture simmer for about 10 minutes, stirring occasionally and breaking down the fruit pieces.

3 After 10 minutes, remove the saucepan from heat and continue to mash the pieces until the mixture reaches the desired consistency.

4 Add the chia seeds and let the mixture cool. The jam will begin to thicken with the chia seeds.

5 Store the jam in the fridge for about 3 hours or overnight for the best results.

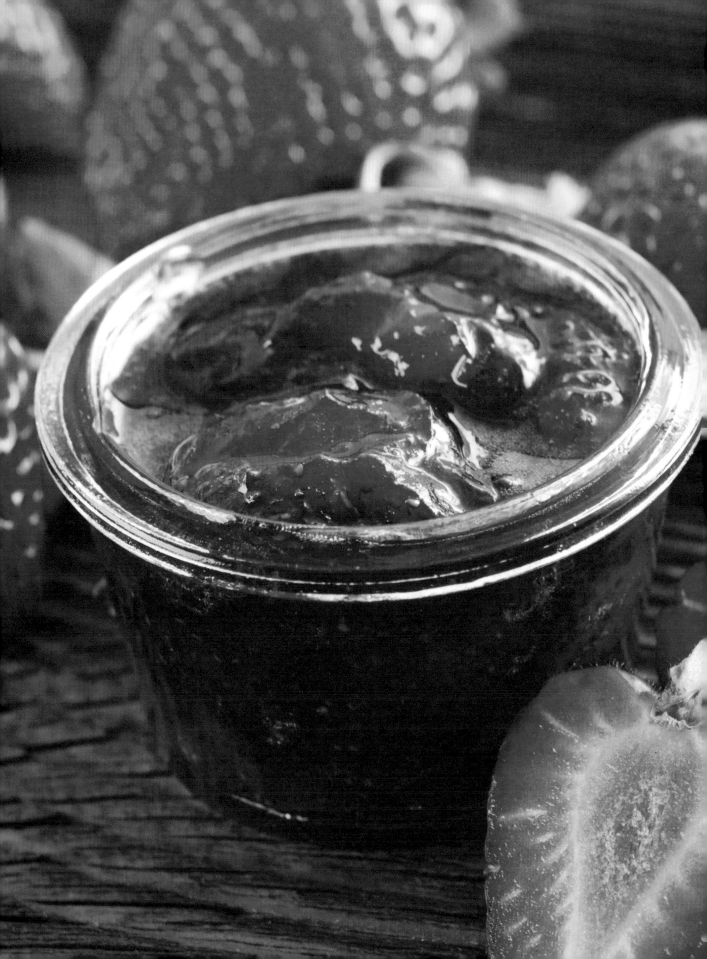

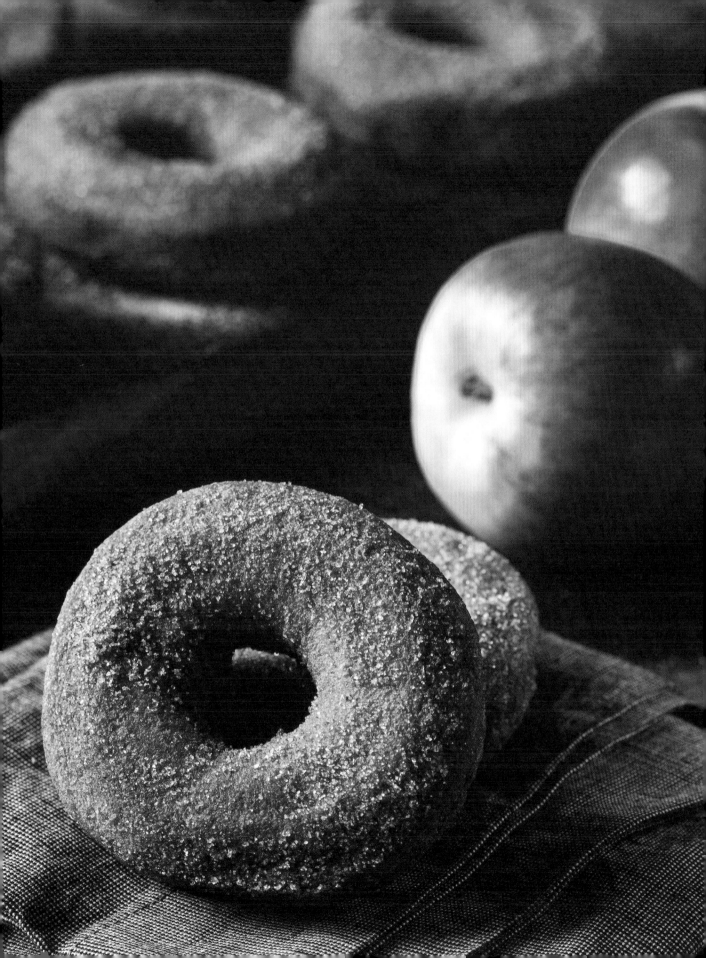

Fall In Love Gluten-Free Donuts

You'll fall in love with these gluten-free donuts that will remind you of autumn any time of year! Not only are these donuts delicious and easy to make, the recipe bypasses all of the sugar (and subsequent inflammation) that comes with eating a more traditional donut.

INGREDIENTS

1½ cups almond flour

⅓ cup Lakanto Golden Monkfruit Sweetener

2 teaspoons apple pie spice

Pinch or ⅛ teaspoon ground nutmeg

Pinch of sea salt

1½ teaspoons baking powder

3 whole pasture-raised eggs

3 tablespoons cinnamon applesauce

1 tablespoon melted ghee

Coconut cooking spray

INSTRUCTIONS

1 Preheat oven to 350°F.

2 In one bowl mix the flour, sweetener, spices, and baking powder.

3 In another bowl, mix the eggs, applesauce, and ghee.

4 Combine the contents of both bowls and mix until well combined.

5 Spay a donut pan with coconut cooking spray and spoon the mixture evenly into the donut spaces.

6 Bake for about 15 minutes or until an inserted toothpick comes out clean. Let them cool for about 10 minutes before popping the donuts out.

Crunchy Bottom Coffee Bundt Cake

Who doesn't love a delicious slice of coffee cake to go along with a nice cup of coffee in the morning? This recipe eliminates the refined sugar, thus reducing potential inflammatory responses and blood sugar imbalances. This coffee cake is made with anti-inflammatory ingredients that give your body the quality fats, carbohydrates, and proteins it needs to stay satisfied and avoid sugar cravings.

INGREDIENTS

Cake

12 pitted dates, chopped

4 egg whites

2 whole pasture-raised eggs

1 cup unsweetened applesauce

1 teaspoon pure vanilla extract

8 scoops grass-fed collagen peptides

½ cup almond flour

⅓ cup coconut flour

3 teaspoons baking powder

½ teaspoon salt

1 teaspoon cinnamon

Coconut cooking spray

Continued...

INSTRUCTIONS

1 Preheat oven to 350°F.

2 Add the dates, egg whites, eggs, applesauce, and vanilla extract to a food processor or blender and pulse until the dates break down into very small pieces.

3 Add the collagen peptides, almond flour, coconut flour, baking powder, salt, and cinnamon and pulse until combined.

4 In a separate bowl, add the topping ingredients and mix until combined.

5 Coat a Bundt pan with coconut cooking spray and add the batter. Sprinkle topping mixture on cake batter and place the pan in the oven.

6 Bake for about 25 to 30 minutes or until an inserted toothpick comes out clean.

7 Once finished baking, let the cake cool for about 10 minutes.

8 Flip cake into a plate and serve immediately.

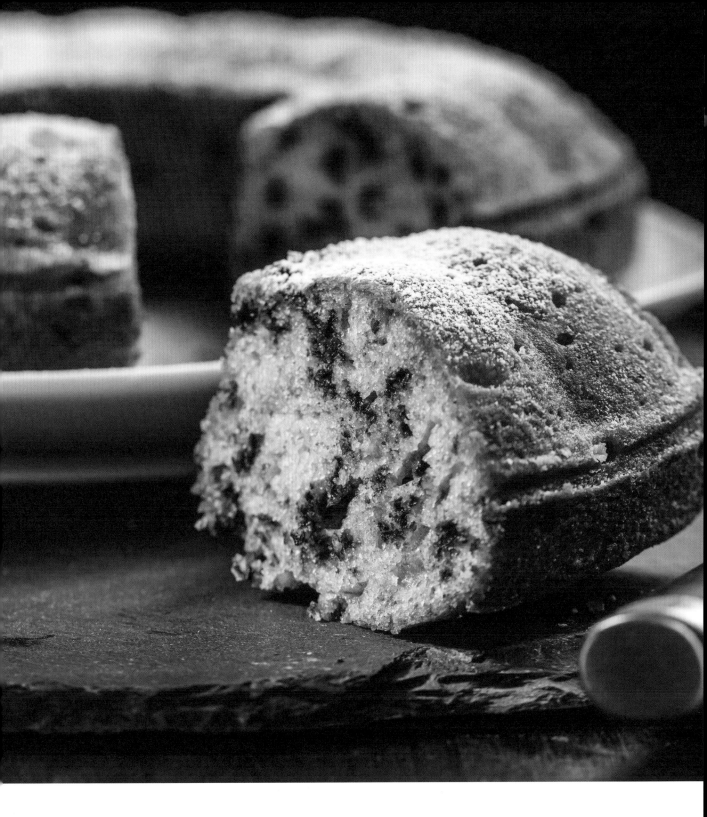

Topping
⅓ cup finely chopped
pecans

3 tablespoons Lakanto Golden
Monkfruit Sweetener

¼ teaspoon cinnamon

¼ teaspoon allspice

¼ teaspoon salt

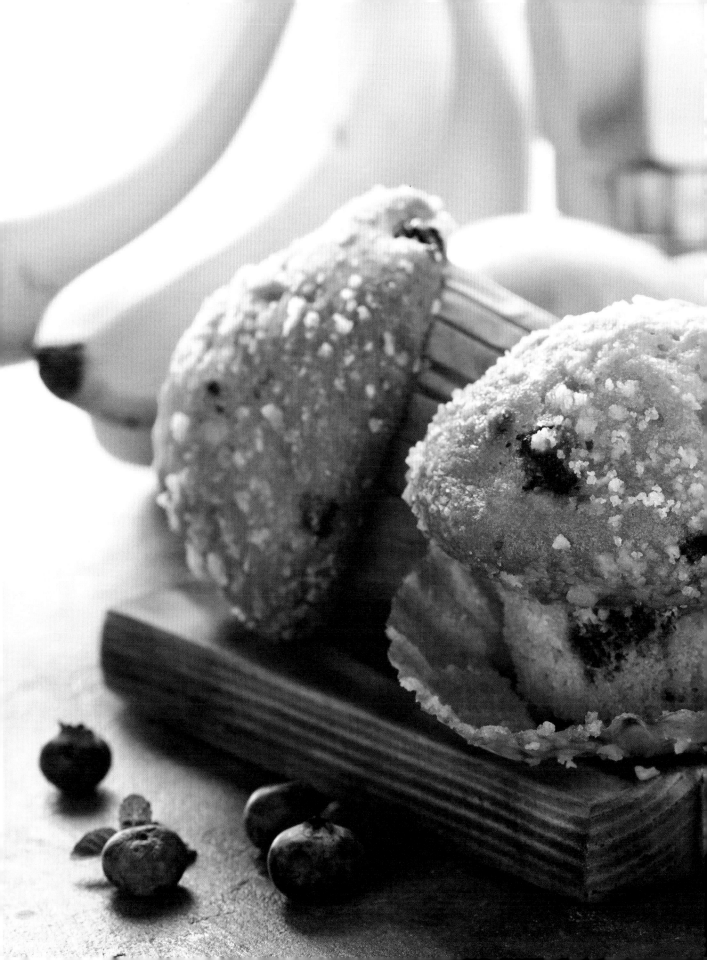

PBJB Breakfast Muffins

These muffins are a great breakfast option thanks to quality fats, carbs, and proteins that will keep you full throughout the morning, as well as combat any snack cravings for inflammatory foods. Blueberries also contain antioxidants and flavonoids called anthocyanins that help your body fight and reduce inflammation for optimal health.

INGREDIENTS

1 cup gluten-free old-fashioned rolled oats

2 ripe medium bananas

2 whole pasture-raised eggs

½ cup non-dairy milk

2 tablespoons raw honey

1 tablespoon melted coconut oil

1½ teaspoons baking powder

½ teaspoon baking soda

½ teaspoon vanilla extract

Pinch of sea salt

⅓ cup peanut butter (or substitute almond butter for peanut sensitivities)

1 cup fresh blueberries

INSTRUCTIONS

1 Heat the oven to 375°F.

2 Place all ingredients except the nut butter and berries into a large food processor or blender and blend until the mix is well combined and halfway smooth.

3 Open the processor or blender lid and add the nut butter. Blend until the mixture is completely smooth.

4 Open the lid and stir in the blueberries.

5 Pour the batter into a greased or lined 12-cup muffin pan.

6 Bake for about 20 minutes or until an inserted toothpick comes out clean. Remove the pan from the oven and let the muffins cool.

Zucchini Banana Nut Muffins

These delicious muffins are great to make when you don't know what else to do with the ripe zucchinis and extra bananas you have on hand. This recipe also uses walnuts, which are rich in omega-3 fatty acids that help keep any inflammation in your body at bay.

INGREDIENTS

2 medium zucchinis, shredded

½ teaspoon sea salt

1 cup almond flour

½ cup coconut flour

½ cup Lakanto Golden Monkfruit Sweetener

1 tablespoon baking powder

⅓ cup walnuts, chopped

1 tablespoon cinnamon

¼ teaspoon nutmeg

Continued...

INSTRUCTIONS

1   Heat oven to 350°F.

2   Shred the zucchini and place it in a strainer. Sprinkle the zucchini with salt and let it rest for about 10 minutes.

3   Transfer the zucchini to a thick paper towel and squeeze out any remaining liquid. You want the zucchini to be dry.

4   In a separate bowl, mix the flours, sweetener, baking powder, nuts, and spices.

5   In another bowl, mix the eggs, mashed bananas, butter or ghee, applesauce, zucchini, and vanilla.

6   Slowly mix the wet and dry ingredients until well combined.

7   Pour the mixture into a greased or lined 12-cup muffin pan and place the pan into the oven for about 20 to 25 minutes or until an inserted toothpick comes out clean.

8   Remove the pan from the oven and let the muffins cool.

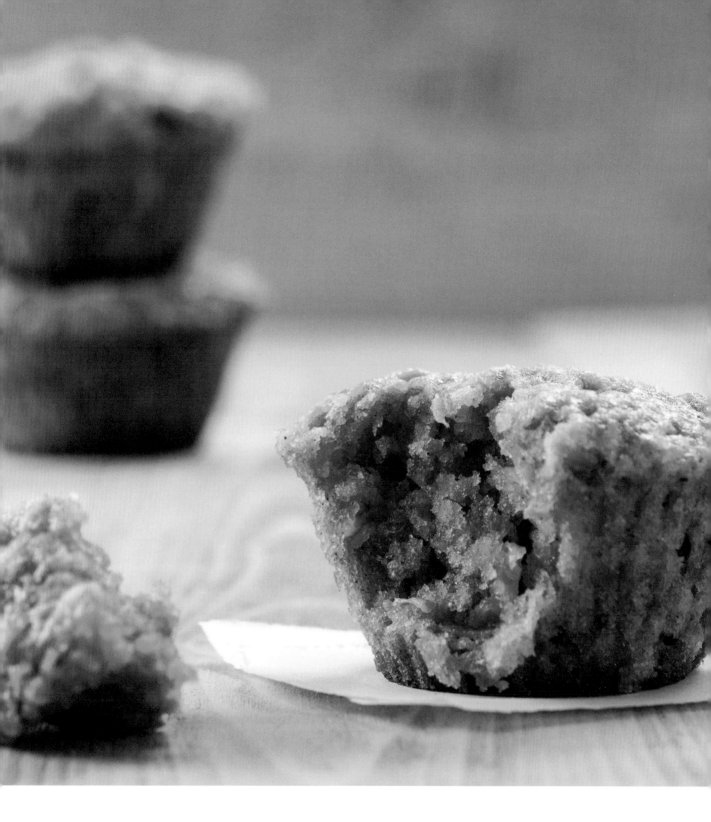

2 whole pasture-raised eggs

2 ripe medium bananas, mashed

⅓ cup or about 5 tablespoons melted grass-fed butter or ghee

⅓ cup unsweetened apple sauce

1 teaspoon vanilla extract

Cranberry Walnut Pumpkin Bread

This bread is a great source of fiber thanks to the pumpkin, almond flour, and coconut flour. The walnuts also provide anti-inflammatory omega-3 fatty acids and the cranberries have anthocyanins which help reduce inflammation and protect against chronic disease.

INGREDIENTS

1 cup canned pumpkin puree

¼ cup pure maple syrup

¼ cup melted ghee

4 large whole pastured-raised eggs, whisked

1 teaspoon pure vanilla extract

1 cup almond flour

¼ cup coconut flour

1 teaspoon baking soda

½ teaspoon baking powder

¼ teaspoon salt

1 teaspoon nutmeg

1 teaspoon allspice

½ teaspoon ground nutmeg

½ teaspoon ground ginger

2 teaspoons ground cinnamon

½ cup dried cranberries

⅓ cup walnuts, chopped

Cooking spray

INSTRUCTIONS

1 Preheat the oven to 350°F.

2 In one bowl, mix the pumpkin puree, maple syrup, ghee, whisked eggs, and vanilla extract. In a separate bowl, mix the dry ingredients.

3 Add the wet ingredients into the dry ingredients bowl and mix well.

4 Grease a 9 x 5-inch loaf pan with cooking spray and place the dough mixture into the pan.

Continued...

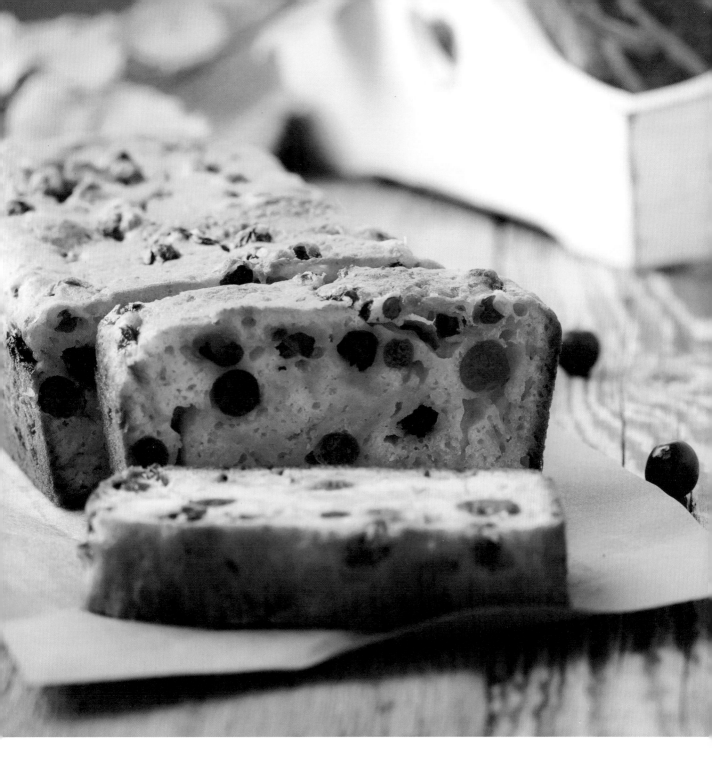

5 Bake in the oven for about 45 to 55 minutes or until the center is firm. If you insert a clean butter knife and it comes out clean, the bread is done.

6 Remove the bread from the oven and allow it to cool for about 20 minutes in the pan.

7 After allowing the bread to cool, flip the bread pan onto a clean plate or cutting board. Wait until the bread is completely cool before you start cutting.

Chocolate Cranberry Protein Balls

If you want to satisfy your sweet tooth without compromising your nutrition goals, this is the snack for you. Coconut contains medium-chained triglycerides that can reduce inflammatory responses within your body. Dark chocolate also has anti-inflammatory compounds that perform similar functions, and collagen peptides are rich in glycine.

INGREDIENTS

1 cup shredded coconut, unsweetened

1 cup almond flour

¾ cup smooth or crunchy almond butter (or nut butter of choice)

3 tablespoons maple syrup

1 teaspoon pure vanilla extract

3 scoops Primal Kitchen Unflavored Collagen Peptides (or collagen flavor of choice)

¼ cup chopped almonds

¼ cup mini dark chocolate chips (if you can't find mini chips, roughly chop up regular-sized chips)

¼ cup dried cranberries

¼ cup water

INSTRUCTIONS

1 Combine all ingredients except the water in a mixing bowl.

2 Using clean hands, combine all the ingredients while slowly adding water little by little until a dough-like mixture forms. It's important to add water a little at a time, as you might not need all of it.

3 Once the dough is formed, break apart pieces of the dough and roll into balls, however large or small you would like them to be. Store them in the fridge for about 30 minutes before serving.

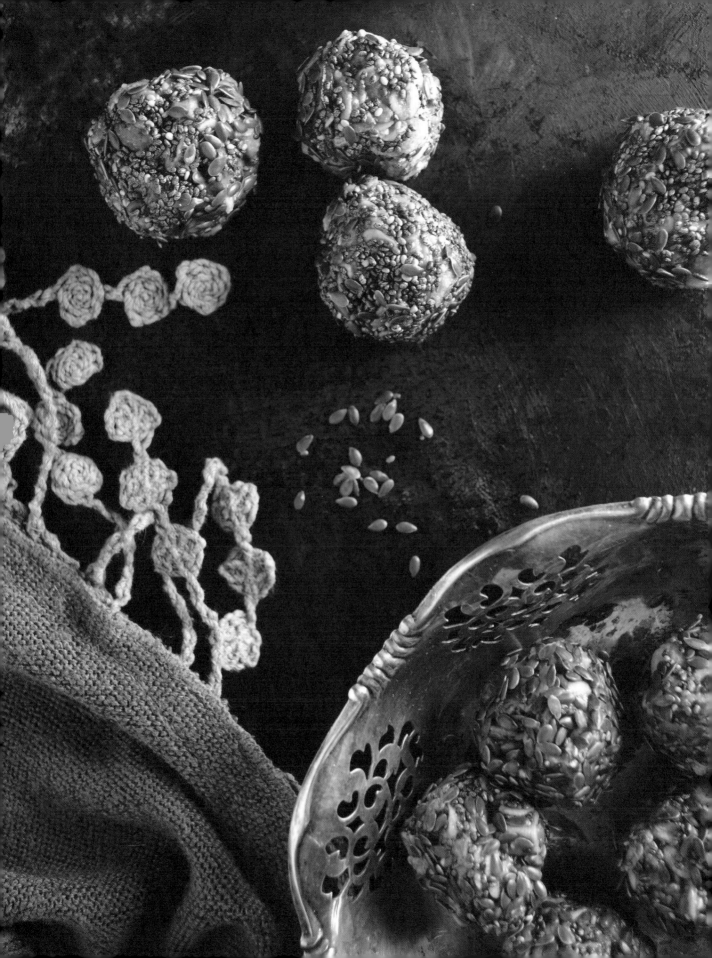

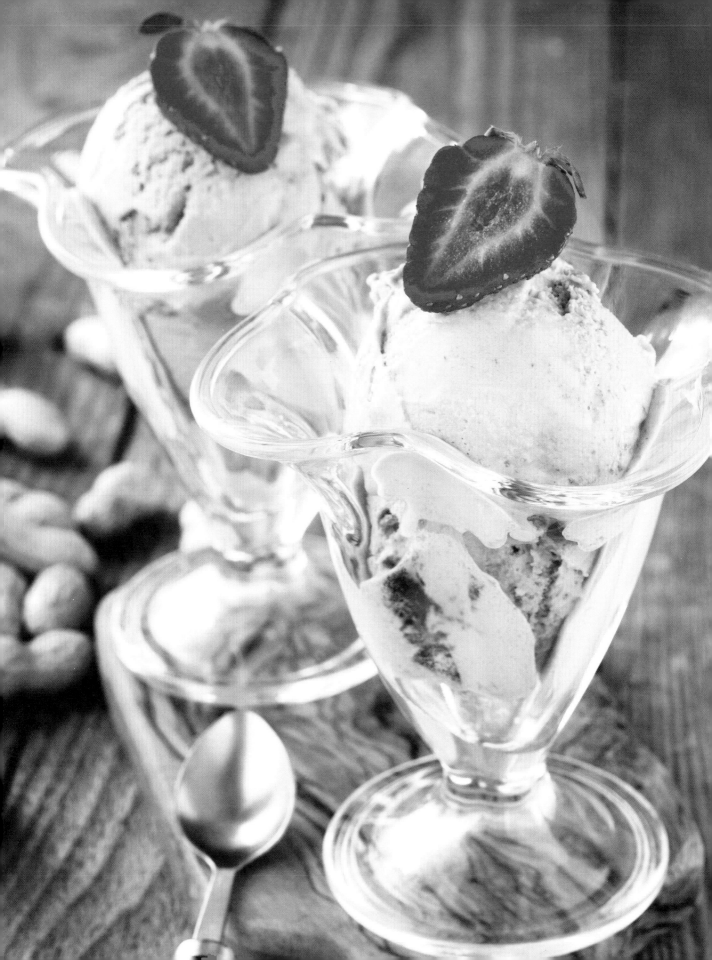

Peanut Butter & Jelly Ice Cream

We all love ice cream, but we could live without the discomfort, bloating, and aches we get after eating dairy. Here is a recipe for ice cream that you can enjoy without any worries. If you have an allergy to peanuts, you can substitute the peanut butter for almond butter.

INGREDIENTS

4 frozen bananas, cut into 4 pieces

½ cup unsweetened non-dairy milk of choice

½ cup peanut butter

1 cup fresh strawberries

2 teaspoons vanilla extract

INSTRUCTIONS

1 Add the frozen bananas and non-dairy milk to a food processor. Set the processor on low, stopping intermittently to scrape the sides of the bowl. Continue to process until smooth.

2 Add the peanut butter, strawberries, and vanilla extract. Process until smooth and the ingredients are incorporated.

3 Pour the mixture into a freezer-safe container and place the container in the freezer for 6 hours or overnight before serving.

METRIC CONVERSIONS

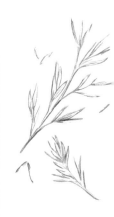

U.S. Measurement	Approximate Metric Liquid Measurement	Approximate Metric Dry Measurement
1 teaspoon	5 ml	5 g
1 tablespoon or ½ ounce	15 ml	14 g
1 ounce or ⅛ cup	30 ml	29 g
¼ cup or 2 ounces	60 ml	57 g
⅓ cup	80 ml	76 g
½ cup or 4 ounces	120 ml	113 g
⅔ cup	160 ml	151 g
¾ cup or 6 ounces	180 ml	170 g
1 cup or 8 ounces or ½ pint	240 ml	227 g
1½ cups or 12 ounces	350 ml	340 g
2 cups or 1 pint or 16 ounces	475 ml	454 g
3 cups or 1½ pints	700 ml	680 g
4 cups or 2 pints or 1 quart	950 ml	908 g

INDEX

219

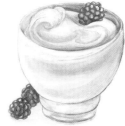

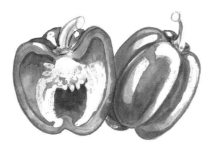

About the Author

Krissy Carbo is a credentialed Registered Dietitian with a Master's degree specializing in integrative and functional approaches to optimal health. After several years practicing as a clinical dietitian and living with an autoimmune disorder caused by chronic inflammation, Carbo learned that nutrient-dense whole foods are essential for reducing inflammation and avoiding many of the common health complications seen today. Carbo launched her private practice, Better With Carbo, where she helps clients identify the root cause of their symptoms and develop achievable nutritional goals. *The Anti-Inflammatory Cookbook* was created to show that nutritious meals don't have to be—and shouldn't be—complicated and that better health is just one meal away.

About Cider Mill Press Book Publishers

Good ideas ripen with time. From seed to harvest, Cider Mill Press brings fine reading, information, and entertainment together between the covers of its creatively crafted books. Our Cider Mill bears fruit twice a year, publishing a new crop of titles each spring and fall.

CIDER MILL PRESS

"Where Good Books Are Ready for Press"

Visit us online at
cidermillpress.com

or write to us at
PO Box 454
12 Spring St.
Kennebunkport, Maine 04046

BOOK PUBLISHERS

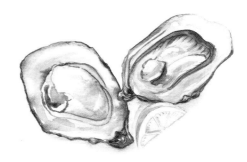

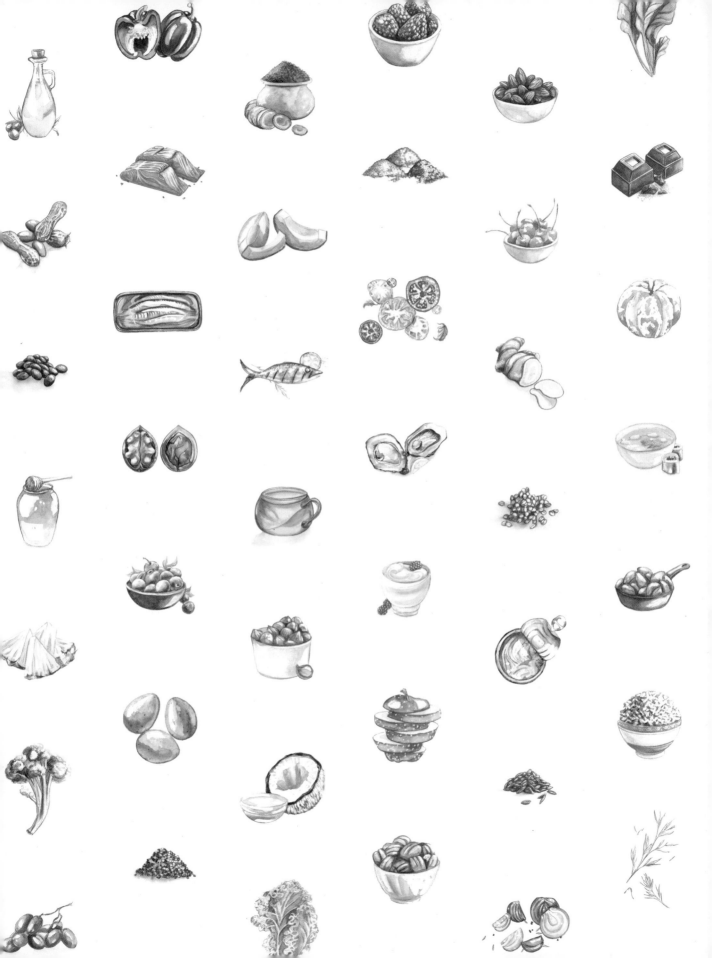

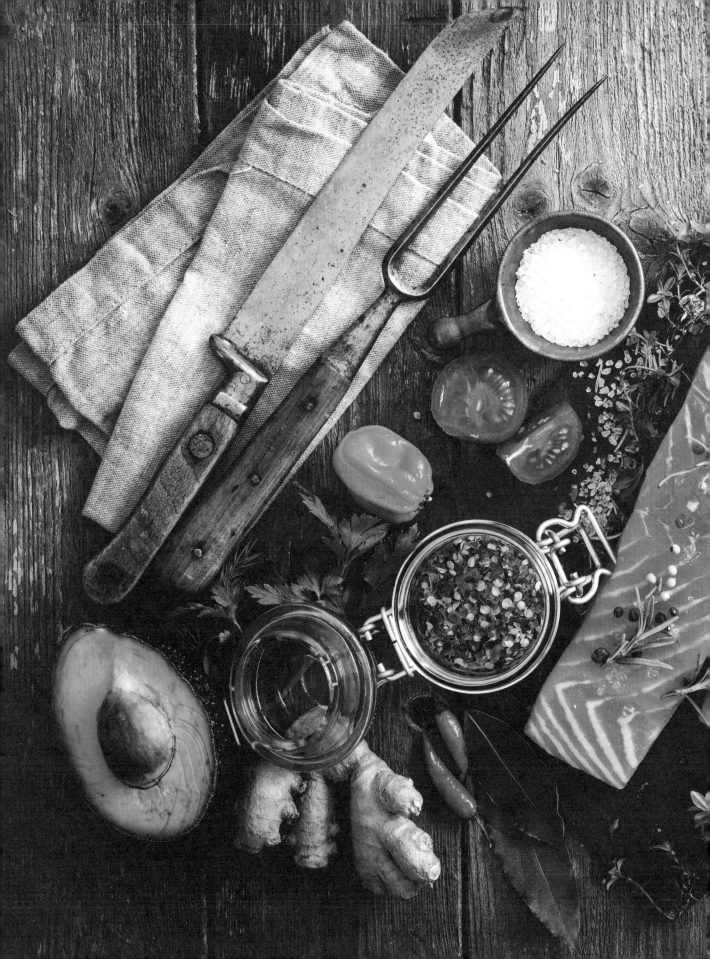